Make Me Laugh
(A Cancer Survival Story)

Jeanine C. Marsters

PublishAmerica
Baltimore

First printing

ISBN: 1-4241-0328-2
PUBLISHED BY
PUBLISHAMERICA, LLLP.
www.publishamerica.com
Baltimore

Printed in the United States of America

Dedication

I dedicate this book to all those battling cancer or any other life-threatening illness. I also dedicate this to my husband Jeff—my hero and my warden, my children Jennifer (and husband Jay), Justin (and his wife Meghan). They are my survival team! I can't leave out the families and friends who are too numerous to name here, you all know who you are. Most of all, I want to dedicate this book to the doctors and nurses who helped me survive and continue to this day. Finally, I dedicate this to Gayle, one of my patients who taught me to fight for life with the strength of a lion.

Introduction

YESTERDAY AS I LEFT WORK ON my way home I noticed the wind blowing. I know that is what the wind does, but hold on. It caught my attention for a different reason. For the first time in several years my hair was actually long enough to blow in the wind. Not a big deal, nothing monumental you say. It sure was to me. It was a sign that my life had returned to normal!

Where do I begin? If you ask my husband he'll tell you I should start at the beginning, just to get the ball rolling so to speak. Interesting as my life was and still is, I never grew up in a log cabin like Abe Lincoln, or did my schoolwork by candlelight like our forefathers. So I'm not sure if the very beginning is where to start.

Have you ever read a story that doesn't seem to get moving until the author can bring his characters in view? Well I have, it is hard to keep a reader's interest. Hold on and bear with me I do think that I have quite a story to tell. It deals with cancer survival. My cancer! My survival! Here we go!

I grew up in the Midwest: Minnesota, Wisconsin, Michigan, and finally Iowa. As a child I traveled a lot, oftentimes feeling like a gypsy. In 1971 I graduated from Duluth East High School, in Duluth, Minnesota. Then on to the big city of Minneapolis, where I worked for one year at IDS (Investors Diversified Services) before entering the United States Navy in December of 1972.

The need to explore the world, to have adventures, came to me one day while doing my job. I talked with a lady I passed by every day on my morning rounds. I was a messenger, fancy title for a mail girl. (Keep in mind I was of course worldly at nineteen, or so I thought.) When I asked her how long she had worked for the company, she surprised me when she said ten years. The thing that made the biggest impression on me was she told me that she started three desks back from where she sat now. Whoa! This was not going to be me! She must have been all of twenty-eight, not married, no children, to a worldly nineteen-year-old, she was old and her life was over, right?

Solution? Join the Navy. Why Navy you ask? It's only because I liked the hats! The traditional naval hat or "cover," as it is called in the military, is a bucket hat (never quite sure why they called it that). Nevertheless I thought they were cool. The hat was basically white with navy blue felt-like trim. The blue trim bordered the hat all the way around coming to a crisscross in the back. It had an insignia pinned on the front, a gold anchor with a rope twisted around it. To me it was just too cute.

The other reason for my choice was that all of the recruiters for the other branches of service were out of their offices the day I stopped by. So the Navy won. I knew that if I didn't go in and see someone at that precise moment I would've lost my nerve and left, never to return.

I served my country for five years as a hospital corpsman. What is a hospital corpsman? She/he is usually the only medical aide that a Marine receives while out in the field, albeit combat or peacetime training. They can also be found in naval hospitals or on board ships. They are not nurses, nor are they doctors. I guess you could say they are a jack-of-all-trades and a master of none. Simply hoping that the sixteen weeks of training she/he receives will be sufficient enough to save a life in time of war. Bill Cosby

6

was a hospital corpsman when he was in the service. On some of the albums I have he often joked about the training he received. Funny yes, but an accurate description of what it was really like during wartime.

It was in the Navy that I met and married my husband Jeff, at the Philadelphia Naval Hospital Chapel. The hospital was imploded a few years ago, a cutback on military spending I guess. Or perhaps they needed to put up a parking lot! So much history gone, not to mention the history of our family beginnings, simply reduced to nothing in the blink of an eye.

Jeff grew up in New England, Maine, to be exact. This should clue you into the fact that it has been interesting combining a New Englander with a Midwesterner. They are areas of the same country but culturally quite different. He was raised on seafood and swam in the ocean. I, on the other hand, was raised on beef and swam in the Great Lakes. This isn't the only difference but you get the picture without my going much further, right?

Our daughter Jennifer was born in January 1978 at the same Naval Hospital Jeff and I were married at. See what I mean about history. Once I got pregnant I opted to discharge. At one time it was a mandatory thing that if you were pregnant you were automatically discharged. The new and modern Navy allowed this to be your choice. Jeff still had about two years left on his enlistment. When Jennifer was two weeks old Jeff was transferred to sunny California where he finished his enlistment as a corpsman with the Marines at Camp Pendleton.

Once discharged, we moved to the Midwest, Iowa to be exact because, my parents lived here. In 1979 the economy wasn't fairing well in New England and jobs were hard to come by. It has been said that once you are out of the service, if you can last one year by finding employment, a place to live, etc. the chance of your needing to return to the military for a sense of security is slim.

We saw many of our friends not make it on the "outside." They had to re-enlist just to take care of their families. By God we were determined we would be counted among those that made it.

You are trained to function well in all facets of the military. The only drawback, it is in the military. With no licenses for many positions you are trained for on the "outside," where do you go? Not much call for tank drivers in civilian life.

Most of the people who you graduated from high school with had gone on to college, gotten married and had started their families. Usually, they were established in various jobs and had their own homes. All you had to your credit was serving your COUNTRY. Sad but true, it leaves you feeling a bit displaced. That along with the fact that this was the time of the Viet Nam War and we all remember how the country felt about the military during that time. Service Personnel were not exactly warmly received in some places. There wasn't the same feeling as when the soldiers came marching home again in WWII. At this time soldiers were considered to be baby killers and their peers were burning the flag not rallying around it.

I was stationed at Great Lakes when the first of the POWs came home. It definitely left quite an impression on me. Even now those images are still vivid in my mind. These were survivors! And it spoke to me in volumes deep in my soul; it also taught me about being a survivor.

Shortly after coming to Iowa our son Justin was born, September of 1980. He is the only true Iowan in the group. During the next five years we lived a somewhat normal life, what exactly is the definition of normal? Do you know? "Usual, conforming to an accepted standard," this is what Webster says. I stayed home and tended our little family, while Jeff went off to work bringing home the bacon. It all sounds fairly typical, doesn't it? Unfortunately, I started to relate to adults on a child's level, you know where Big Bird, Bert and Ernie and Mr. Rogers are your best friends. I am so glad there weren't any giant purple dinosaurs around at that time; I don't think I could have handled it.

It was in the fall of 1985 that I decided to use my GI Bill to get an education, why not I had earned it. Jeff and I were in one of the last group of enlistees that had earned an education

8

allotment just by enlisting in one branch of the service or another. In the 1980s the government decided to give us ten years to use our education allotments or lose them. Not knowing what to study I started out in general education, the basics, "Fundamentals of Math" for example. It had been so long that I was in school I needed to know how to add one and one all over again. It still equals two, doesn't it?

Eventually I received my associate degree in both nursing and science. It was not much of a surprise to my maternal grandmother who always said when I was a little girl I wanted to be a nurse. Oh, really, I thought. Anyhow, this is where my story truly begins...

Disclosure

Names of certain individuals in *Make Me Laugh* have been changed to protect their privacy.

Chapter One

IN HIS BOOK, PUBLISHED IN 1956, *The Stress of Life,* Hans Selye, a researcher in psychosomatic medicine defines stress as "the rate of wear and tear within the body as it adapts to change or threat." *Mosby's Medical Dictionary* states that stress, "is an adverse condition during which we may experience tension or fatigue, feel unpleasant emotions, and sometimes develop a sense of hopelessness or futility."

Stress puts you in the "flight or fight" mode. First, stress hormones including adrenaline and cortisol flood the body, causing:

*your body's need for oxygen to increase
*your heart rate and blood pressure to go up
*the blood vessels in your skin to constrict
*your muscles to tense
*your blood sugar level to increase
*your blood to have an increased tendency to clot
*your body's cells to pour stored fat into the bloodstream

All of this puts strain on your heart and the lining of your arteries, so much that if you already have coronary artery disease, stress might make you experience chest pain, which is called angina. The increased tendency for the blood to clot may cause some people to develop a clot in their arteries, which could cause a heart attack.

The tendency for your bowel and intestinal muscles to constrict, are due to a sudden release of adrenaline, which can lead to stomach problems. In addition, the release of adrenaline can precipitate a number of mental illnesses, but it can activate these diseases of the brain to those who may already be prone to them.

FACTS

*Almost nine out of ten adults have experienced serious stress in their lives.

*More than four out of ten adults suffer adverse health affects from stress.

*Seventy-five to ninety percent of all doctor's office visits are for stress related complaints.

*Working mothers, in particular, are among the people most likely to experience stress.

*Symptoms of stress include irritability; sleep disturbances, appetite changes, muscle tension, apathy, fatigue, headache and frequent illness.

*Stress can be brought about by external factors such as conflicts in relationships, pressures, and even traffic.

*Internal factors—such as a desire for perfection, feeling of helplessness, blaming yourself for things that are out of your control or intense worry—can also cause stress.

I am sure you are wondering where exactly I plan on going with all of this information. Why did I tell you about it? I believe in the deepest part of my soul that stress has played an important part of my struggle with cancer. As I show you the facts, you could have put my name in front of each condition. I have experienced all of the above symptoms at one point or another.

At the time I made my decision to go into nurses training, Jeff and I were in the throws of simply raising our little family. We were as close to the 1950s TV show *Leave it to Beaver* as you could be in the 1980s. Talking to people, mostly women, of my generation I have discovered that most of us have tried to model our families after the Cleavers. That was an era where life seemed simple. June Cleaver was the perfect mother and wife.

Unfortunately the 1980s were a different time and women were putting undue stress on themselves trying to become that perfect family where both mom and dad worked. What wasn't included in the script was the fact that it wasn't real. There wasn't any Cleaver family, a perfect family where Ward went off to work while June stayed at home and baked cookies, tended the children in a full costume of jewelry, dresses and fresh makeup all the time.

I was at a point in my personal life that I desperately wanted to reconnect with the real world again. I wanted to be known for my own achievements not just as the children's mother, my husband's wife, or my parents' daughter. I wanted to be able to give something of myself to the world, to society. So by using my benefit allotment from the military, I was able to obtain my nursing degree. We have a two-year college not far from my home and they offered a two-year Registered Nurse program. June Cleaver never would have done that, would she?

After graduating in May of 1988, I immediately started studying for my NCLEX nursing boards. This I found was the worst test of human endurance that I had ever encountered. Or so I thought, then I spoke to some of the doctors I worked with about their medical boards. They suffered far more than I did. The mental anguish I put myself and my family through was awful. Spending countless hours, days and weeks poring over my many review books.

Then added to this, practicing my new skills as a GN (Graduate Nurse). End result of all the torture was to receive a

Registered Nurse (RN) license that September. A license that gave me permission to clean up the three "p"s (pee, poop, and puke), think about that for a minute. When you consider that every woman is a nurse at heart. Mothers have been nursing for years without a license. Is that legal?

It simply is about the female/maternal instinct our gender possesses. It is in our nature to care for others. According to Philip Gold, MD, Chief of the National Institutes of Health Clinics Neuroendocrine Branch, "It appears that women have an innate stress system that are exquisitely sensitive, to enhance their ability to care give throughout life." Before I get in trouble with the male nurses in the group, I will add that some men have gotten in touch with their nurturing side too and have made wonderful contributions to the art of nursing.

The only downside to our ability to plan and care for others is that often we rarely apply this to ourselves. This skill requires learning how to develop limits and boundaries; we rarely find time to take care of ourselves. Nursing School did not prepare me for that. There were so many ill people out there I didn't have time to think of myself and take care of them. The answer I give to you now is "honey, you better make time." Even fifteen minutes to connect to yourself will be better for you than keeping the doctor away with the proverbial "apple a day."

I discovered the real world of nursing after school. It didn't mean one-on-one patient care as I was used to in my clinical experiences as a student nurse. The ratio of nurse to patients in the real world, in 1988, was more like ten of them to one of me. Trying to manage patient care, medication administration, treatments, IV therapy and charting on ten patients wasn't going to be easy. Perhaps a course in juggling would have been more helpful. This ratio has dropped significantly in the years that followed. The nurses had fewer patients, but the ones they were assigned to are much sicker. The people wait longer before they seek out medical assistance. This makes their conditions much more complicated than back when I graduated.

In school they taught us about communicating with the

patients on a more personal level, using our well-choreographed therapeutic communication skills. This got tossed out the window right at the start. Who had time to talk to their patients when you were now taking care of ten of them? As you exited each patient's room you mumbled your name followed by "I will be your nurse tonight." Simply praying that no one called you back to answer any questions. I learned to adapt quickly though using the old "sink or swim" method, from the school of hard knocks. I was ready for the funny farm as well as the circus. I had learned how to juggle. Hooray for me!

In "new millennium" nursing there are dry eraser boards in each patient rooms, this is where the staff caring for the patient writes their names on at the beginning of their shift. This takes us even farther away from bedside nursing. I never have figured out for sure if the boards were for the nurses or the patients. Maybe for the nurse in a way to help her remember if she was in the right room. Or for the patients so in case it's four or five hours that you were in to see them (that is what patients always tells you). When in actuality it may have been only thirty minutes since you were in to check on them. I can attest personally to the fact that you lose all sense of time and space when you are a patient in the hospital before she/he sees her/his nurse they know who to complain about and to whom. The only drawback that I see is that I now need to find the time to write my name on the board. Sound familiar? *"I'm late; I'm late for a very important date. No time to say hello good-bye, I'm late, I'm late, I'm late!* Isn't that what the white rabbit said to Alice? It isn't just a fairy tale anymore? It's reality!

I believe that the lack of nurses at the bedside has been a bone of contention since the time of Florence Nightingale. Now there was an example of a true nurse. She was able to be at the bedside to really care for her patients. She would hold their hands; write letters home for them, as well as caring for their wounds. With the added paperwork that is expected of the "new millennium" nursing staff there isn't much time to spend with the patients anymore.

The patients are coming to the hospital sicker than before and insurance dictates how long they can stay there. I am sure Florence is rolling over in her grave thinking that we have become paperwork junkies, in a paperwork junky world. Or nowadays we are connected to technology. We do our charting on computer, use PDAs for medication passing and carry cell phones to answer call lights. So, what are next roller blades? What would happen if somebody pulled the plug?

A prime example, my medical insurance always sends a form out each time they review a claim sent into them. It wasn't too long ago that I received ninety-six individual envelopes (they didn't even fit in the mailbox). Couple this with the cost of ninety-six separate stamps, which by the way added up to twenty-six dollars. Seems to me that they could've saved everyone a lot of hassle by putting them all in one envelope. Hmm?

At this same time another stressor came into my life in an all too different package. Five foot two, eyes of brown, and commonly known in our family as MOM (to those nurses out there this is not the acronym for milk of magnesia). She had an argument with her husband, my stepfather, and then came to my home seeking refuge. Lucky for her it was Jeff answering the door (I was of course at work) or I would have sent her home to try to work things out. It wasn't like they had never argued before. It had been like this for most of their nearly thirty-year relationship.

My brother, sister and I have gone through those years of chaos with them and rarely batted an eye when they were "at it again." But Jeff was not familiar with the pattern. He didn't know anyone that had such a turbulent relationship as they did. At least not until now that is. As the years have gone on in our twenty-eight plus years of marriage he has seen examples of this now in his own family.

I love my mother very much. Over the years as adults you could say we have become more like friends. Still you know what they say about visiting relatives, well when it is your mother and your husband's mother-in-law, you get the picture? Her overnight stay lasted eight months. One can never go home again, at least not as an adult, albeit parent or child.

Jeff and my mother had built a tolerable relationship back then; it has grown more as the years pass by. My mother says he is more like a son than a son-in-law. And Jeff thinks of her as another mother. And guess who became the go-between or shall I say the ping-pong ball in their lives? For me it was nearly impossible because all of my life I had learned to internalize my emotions. A great big bundle of pent-up raw nerves is what I was like most of the time. Taking it all personally. Always trying to please everyone.

I was working the evening shift, from three to eleven. This became my refuge. I found myself volunteering to work on my days off to avoid the tension at home. It was only the tension that I brought on myself. The pay was great but the toll on my mind and body was not. I am talking about the immune system. Stress also causes the immune system to not function properly, which enables you to catch every nasty bug out there.

In psychological circles this would be known as *avoidance behavior*, always running and hiding from things. Never willing to face anything head-on. If you can avoid it, you will never have to deal with it, right? I needed to be able to tell them both how I felt, but for some reason I couldn't. I had learned too young that in order to keep peace in life you never rocked the boat. I found out much later that this could be a self-destructive behavior.

At Christmas of the same year I was touched deeply by a young girl of twenty-six who had what seemed to be an incurable illness. We became not only patient and nurse, but also friends. I will never forget her face; it is etched in my brain forever. She had the largest brown eyes I had ever seen, with brown shoulder length hair. She reminded me of Pebbles, freckle-faced with her ponytail on top of her head secured in a rubber band we found in the desk at the nurse's station. She had become quite frail from her illness, barely weighing ninety-five pounds. Yet, she was lovely to me.

I would request to be her nurse for many days in a row. We both laughed and cried together. Even though I say she was frail she had the strength of a lion. She was a fighter. She fought her illness to the end. It was the time I spent with her that taught me

17

how to fight with the strength of a lion, at that time not knowing I would need these lessons all too soon.

I can remember, during my annual physical, my doctor asked me how I was doing. I simply burst into tears. When I explained the situation to him at home, my mother living with us and all. He told me I had to stop it. It was not healthy for me and eventually could harm me. Little did I know what the next months had in store for me or perhaps I would have heeded his warning. Wouldn't it be nice sometimes to hold our lives in a crystal ball and see just a glimpse of our future? Or would it?

It was during the Christmas season that Jeff told me he "refused to spend another Christmas like this one." That either my mother went or he did! Thanks, Jeff. If my memory serves me right it was you that allowed her to stay in the first place. I would've sent her back home the day she came. Now he was giving me the problem to deal with.

In January, I found myself tiring easier and getting sore throats more frequently. Naturally I attributed this to my hectic work schedule. Never having my tonsils out, I was all too familiar with tonsillitis in the winter months. I battled this ailment all through my childhood and as an adult. So I thought! I should have remembered that the biblical quote was only physician heal thyself not nurse heal thyself. Here I was trying to diagnose and treat myself. I didn't like to see doctors for myself. I avoided them at all costs. This seems a little quirky to me, a nurse who doesn't like doctors?

Jeff and I decided that we needed to get away. We needed a rest. We asked my mother if she could watch the children while we went to Minneapolis for a weekend with another couple. You are probably thinking that it would not be an issue for her to watch the children. Normally not, but early in their lives she told Jeff and I she was not going to be a baby-sitter for us. If we wanted to go anywhere and do anything we had to hire our own sitter, she was not going to do it. To this day I believe that was the only time we ever asked her, although she did volunteer fairly often.

It was during the Minneapolis trip that I showed my friend (who is also a nurse) a weird rash I had found on my chest. Small raised, reddened areas with a silvery hue that just sat there, never growing in size, not itching, no pain, they were just there. She didn't know what to make of them either, but admitted that they were definitely weird.

After our weekend in the Twin Cities, it was all too clear that the pressures I had been under were getting to me. I could feel the tension return when we entered the driveway at home. The first night home I developed a severe toothache. Which after many hours took me out in the middle of the night heading to the emergency room for a shot of *Demerol* to take away the pain. Before going to the emergency room, it was my mother who helped me pace the night away trying to help me deal with the pain. I have discovered that through the years mothers, including mine, had a way of making things better. They seem to have all the answers to whatever ails us.

I don't want to give you the impression that my mother was hard to live with; it was more to do with the situation, all under one roof. None of us were ever able to be totally alone for some needed quiet time. What made it more difficult is that I have never been able to tell anyone my true feelings. So whenever Jeff and my mom disagreed I assumed it was my fault, my problem. Remember that goes way back into my childhood when I believed if you really tell how you feel they went away, sometimes forever.

The next morning I found a dentist in the yellow pages that advertised specializing in the care of chickens, my kind of guy. I had the tooth extracted. I spent the rest of the day in bed napping from all the pacing I did the night before. There was some oozing from the hole left in mouth by the tooth for many hours after. I didn't realize that cancer was already circulating in my body, not allowing me to clot properly after the extraction.

The next puzzle piece in the equation was that one morning while I was in the shower I found bumps on the top of my head. *Enough was enough*, I thought! I called my doctor figuring he would get rid of them, whatever they were. It was a Friday and I was in his office by ten. He agreed with me, the rash was weird; in fact, he told me he "hadn't seen anything like it in all his years of practice." I laughed. I always wanted to be unique, I thought to myself. He gave me a prescription for an antihistamine and sent me on my way, even though he wasn't sure it was an allergic reaction. Giving me explicit instructions to return to the office, or call him the first of the week if the rash did not start to go away. Could he have suspected there was possibly more?

It was the weekend, Jeff and the kids spent most of their time in Charles City at a swim meet (our children were both swimmers). I spent most of the weekend bonding with my couch, nursing yet another sore throat. My mother would frequently run to Wendy's for a frosty, the only thing that seemed to soothe my throat. I was so tired and weak. I was afraid my mononucleosis was back. I had it once while I was under stress during nursing school. There is that nasty word again, it keeps popping up, doesn't it—STRESS.

I learned one thing since that time, sometimes in order to make changes in your life; you could do yourself some good by contracting an illness. Why? Because when you are faced with a life-threatening illness, it gives you enough of a pause to reevaluate your life. It also gives you a sense of freedom, enabling you to head in a different direction.

I knew that I couldn't continue on with what was going on at home, work or relationships. Jeff and his ultimatum, my doctor telling me that I had to end it and my only refuge WORK. My body took over and with a sense of survival in mind, I got sick. Really sick! I am sure that some people do not understand this; it is a hard concept to grasp. I also know that some people will understand all too well that there are times when you don't see any way out of a bad situation.

In the past I had always run away. I ran away from home when I was eighteen because I thought life was too tough there. I didn't know how to talk things out when there was a problem with those I loved. I didn't know that to tell someone my feelings, even negative ones was an all right thing to do. If you rocked the

20

boat too much people around you, who you loved would leave, right? It was always safer for me to hold everything inside. I guess cancer for me was my way of running away again without really leaving home. Remember I ran away to the Navy to avoid winding up in a dead-end job. Running had become my MO (Motive Operandi).

On Monday, I called my doctor as he had ordered, to let him know that my rash was still there. He sounded genuinely concerned and made an appointment for me that afternoon to see a dermatologist. I agreed and showed up promptly at one-thirty as ordered. It was not too clear to the dermatologist as to what he thought I had, but he thought it could be one of two things. Both would be benign in nature. The only way to be sure he told me was to get a biopsy of one of them.

I was led back to another exam room where he injected two of the little devils and proceeded to remove them. Wait a minute! I wasn't clotting! They needed to hold pressure on the area for quite awhile after suturing it closed. When I was well enough to be dismissed, I went directly to the hospital where I was already fifteen minutes late for my shift.

As I put my purse away I noticed that there was blood on my uniform pants, the area on my abdomen was still oozing. I simply slapped another gauze dressing on the spot and secured it tightly. Being a surgical nurse I knew all too well how to apply a pressure dressing, it would stop the oozing and I would be okay. Or would I? Things were suspicious, but not discernible enough to get my attention.

I learned how to survive both from my special patient and by the tragedies I had experienced in my own life. I developed my survival skills at a young age. Those lessons I learned then have fared well through the years. Just as I survived things in my youth, it gives me the opportunity to call myself a cancer survivor today.

You see I lost a brother when I was nine years old, just before the 4th of July. He was six and my other brother was seven. The two of them took the training wheels off of their bicycles and went on a bike ride. That was the last time I saw the younger one. He was hit by a dump truck and was killed. The sad part of the whole thing is that morning I had asked him to go and pick raspberries with me down by the railroad tracks. He said no. He told me he was going biking. I got mad at him and was never able to tell him I was sorry. I have carried that guilt around for many years. In the blink of an eye he was gone.

On July 4 I was to represent the VFW on a float in the local parade. My step-dad was a veteran in the Korean War, so my mom and dad were active members. Oftentimes, I went with them as a junior member of the VFW. That year they had me ride on the float. I was to smile and wave to the people in the crowd. I learned only how to keep a "stiff upper lip" that day. MY English grandparents would be proud.

In those days there was no such thing as counseling. No one ever went into therapy like they do now. It is an unfortunate circumstance, because my brother and I definitely needed it. In fact the whole family could have benefited by a little time on the "old" couch. Know what I mean? Perhaps we could have saved our family. My parents split up over the death of my brother. I think that the split could have been looming in the background but after his death they could not come back together.

It was Christmas of that same year that I lost the only father I had ever known. The step-dad who along the parade route that day I sat on the float telling me to remember to smile. After their split he took my brother to live with him and Mother was left with me. Christmas Eve he was on his way from work to spend Christmas with his sister and brother-in-law. That is where my brother was staying. On his way his car skidded on the ice in the dark and hit a tree. He was killed instantly. There was a lot of turmoil for a long time after that.

The spring of 1964 was when the next tragedy struck our family. My mother was in a car accident and injured pretty severely. During that time my brother and I bounced around a bit. From relative to friends and then finally home. These three episodes taught me that you just keep that "stiff upper lip" and hold it all inside in order to move on. Never having to deal with it all. Because if you don't think about it, you don't have to feel the pain…

Chapter Two

I REMEMBER THE DAY CLEARLY...THE day my world stood still. I was watching the videotape *Lonesome Dove*. Jeff had taped it for me the night before. I was hemming a pair of work pants for him. The date was February 8, 1989...it was cold and sunny outside...the time was 10:30 a.m. when the phone rang. It was my doctor...Remember he had sent me to the dermatologist looking for a diagnosis for the rash I had three days earlier. The silly bumps that once were just a few had now peppered my entire chest and head. Do you know to this day I never have finished watching the movie? Now I have no desire to either.

Jeff and my mom worked for the same company with a gal whose mother once had a rash on her head, her diagnosis turned out to be brain cancer. To her I owe a large debt of gratitude, it was because of her I went to the doctor early on when my rash first appeared on my head.

After the cordial hello, I was startled when the voice asked if I was home alone. I finally realized who the voice belonged to, my doctor. Why did he care if I was alone? I hesitantly told him that I was. His response was that he needed to see Jeff and me in his office as soon as possible.

All I felt was instant panic. My body started to shake. I had a gripping tight feeling in my chest. There was the warm feeling you get from an increase in adrenaline, remember the "fight or flight" response. I learned about this in school. You know what I mean the old "Adrenaline Rush." A wave of nausea also came over me as I held the phone tightly to my ear. I wanted to run away. I hadn't felt that scared in years. Those awful years when I lost the people I loved.

I finally was able to ask him what this was all about. He told me he wouldn't discuss it with me over the phone. I kept pressing him for an answer. Finally, I was able to wear him down. He blurted out that my "biopsy report was back from the pathologist. It showed I had METASTATIC CANCER." I could feel the burning in my eyes as the tears began to well up in them. This is not what I expected. I thought it was something benign. No big deal! How wrong I was.

CANCER, are six letters of the alphabet that sent chills running down your spine as a nurse let alone as a patient. I heard nothing else he said. I somehow agreed to call Jeff and meet with him in his office just as soon as we could.

Once off the phone with the doctor I called Jeff hysterical and managed to heave out the words "I have cancer." I told him he had to come home right now!

Every time I said the word cancer I seemed to choke on it myself. My God what have you done to me? My God am I going to…DIE? So many thoughts kept whirling through my mind in those first moments after I hung up the phone…was I going to die, what would happen to my children, would I go to heaven, who would Jeff remarry? I can't explain why I had those kinds of thoughts, I just did. The more I thought about it the more I got angry…in fact I got DAMN mad! CANCER has always meant a death sentence to others, not for me!

According to *Funk & Wagnall Dictionary*, the definition of anger is: "a feeling of sudden and strong displeasure and antagonism directed against the cause of an assumed wrong or injury." No truer words were ever written than those. I was by

24

this definition really angry. In fact I was downright pissed off! Knowing God as I do, I know that He Himself had gotten angry on many occasions. The Bible is loaded with stories recording the fact. He has also used his anger to motivate some of us stubborn ones to get a job done. I did just that, I found out I could use anger as a tool to help me survive.

It wasn't long before Jeff picked me up…the drive to the doctor's office was a blur. I was numb. I felt like I wasn't in the car with him as we drove through town. I could hear nothing, the songs on the radio, and the hum of the car engine or Jeff sitting quietly next to me fighting back his own tears. I had always believed I was a model citizen and a contributing member of society; we didn't get cancer, did we? Our lives would change now, all that we have known until now would be different. At the time we didn't honestly know how much it would change.

We walked slowly into the clinic building near the hospital. Neither one of us speaking or even looking at each other. Too afraid that if our eyes met even for a moment it would open the floodgate of tears we were both holding back. I kept thinking that if I blinked hard enough it would all go away. Please wake me up, honey; shake me hard to stop this nightmare. It wasn't a dream; it was real life, my life.

A nurse escorted us back into an examination room without delay where we waited for the doctor. I just knew that when he came in he would straighten all of this out, explaining and apologizing for this big mistake. Jeff and I continued to sit in silence as we waited; processing the information we had received thus far, still not able to look at each other.

In nurses training I remember studying about death and dying. Identifying that there are patterns to the dying process: initial shock and disbelief, denial, anger, bargaining, a sense of loss and depression and finally acceptance. Personally I went through all of these steps in my mind as the words "You have cancer" kept reverberating in my ears.

When the doctor came into the exam room I looked at his face searching for a sign, a smile or an apology. Something to

25

signal an error had been made. Nothing. It wasn't wrong! No one made a big boo-boo. It was all true. Again I felt numb.

He started talking about how we needed to find out what kind of cancer it was. All I could think of was, *you mean there are different kinds?* Perhaps I should have paid just a little more attention to the different cancer types in nursing school. I was so afraid of cancer and dying that I listened but I didn't hear anything about the subject when we were studying it. Besides, I am one of those people who mentally contracted all the illnesses I read about so the bad ones I used to skim through in a hurry. Is this hypochondria or normal?

The conversation by then was just between Jeff and the doctor; I paced around the room crying and repeating the words "It isn't true! I can't believe it! It's not fair." Everyone agreed it wasn't fair, but I could see that they weren't going to do anything to change the situation. They weren't making it go away. I finally looked at my doctor and for the first time it hit me I really must have cancer. I could see tears in his eyes along with the strain on his brow. With the softness in his voice he finally convinced me. My God I have cancer! This wasn't so funny.

What do I do now? Where do we go from here? In one split second I made up my mind that I was going to survive, that no matter what it took I would win. I would see my children become adults with children of their own. So let us find out what kind of cancer I have so I can begin the good fight. The fight for my life!

He talked to me about the fact that the skin lesions I had were a secondary cancer. They were not sure where the primary source was. I had a pap smear the month before, so that didn't need to be repeated. My doctor kept sifting through things on the desk while thinking out loud.

I have known him for many years both professionally and as our family doctor so it kind of scared me to see him almost cry. I guess we all get this mistaken impression that our doctors don't feel things like we do. That is a myth I know doctors feel pain too. They hate to be the one to tell a patient about a bad diagnosis or a family that their loved ones had died. To some, they feel that somehow it was their fault, a sense of failure. Sound familiar?

He told us that after all the test results were in he would get back to us later on that day. In any case whether a primary source could be found or not he was sending me to the Mayo Clinic for further evaluation and possible treatment. He explained that they saw things on a much larger scale at Mayo than we did and they would be better equipped to handle this, whatever this is. As we started to leave the exam room he gave me a hug and shook Jeff's hand, reassuring us we would get through this.

I was scheduled to go downstairs to the first floor to have a mammogram. They had gotten a baseline once before about three years earlier when I thought I had discovered a suspicious lump in my breast. So they would be able to compare it easily noticing if there was any difference. If you have never had a mammogram then, my friend, you are truly missing out on one of life's secret little tortures. It reminds me of being put on the rack and being stretched. My breasts already sag. The doctors always write in my history and physical that I have "pendulous" breasts. All I can say is that ever since I have had my first mammogram they are getting longer with each subsequent one.

First, they lead you to a changing room where you place a pink cape around your upper body. Next you remove all deodorant traces with the kind of wipes I used to use on my children's backsides during diaper changes. If you don't remove the deodorant it will interfere with the results of the test somehow is what they tell you. A technician escorts you into the room where the mammogram machine is.

They position you in such a manner that you couldn't believe your body actually does that, but this isn't the worst of it. They pick your breast up placing it on a cold metal plate and firmly compress it with another clear plate. To me, my breast under the glass resembled a pancake with a nipple...get the picture? Torture, right?

Two things crossed my mind at this point. First, it must have been a man who invented this beast. Second I wondered how women who were flat chested managed this little maneuver. One person came to mind immediately; she was about my height but at least one hundred pounds lighter than I was. She wore a size 0 I think, or perhaps it was a -0. We always kidded her about needing only a training bra that she didn't even need a bikini she could get by with two Band-Aids. Somehow the image in my head caused me to crack up. The technician asked me what was so funny, I told her nothing; I was keeping this chuckle to myself. I didn't have to share everything. I've given them my body; my mind would be my own. The only conciliation to the ordeal, was knowing that they often perform mammograms on men.

While they are flattening my breast to about one-quarter inch they had me place my other arm behind my back along with the cape. I felt like Superman, even if I wasn't flying yet, I knew I was preparing for takeoff soon. If you have never experienced this I hope I haven't spooked you into not getting one. I may have exaggerated a little, the discomfort you feel is momentary. The most important thing is that a mammogram may possibly save a life, and that life could be yours.

From there I went to the x-ray department across the street, in the hospital, to schedule my CT scan. We were told they could do it that afternoon. I had to drink three glasses of this liquid, contrast they called it. It would help to see all that is in me and more. It smelled like licorice, but it sure didn't taste like it.

A CT or CAT scan stands for computerized tomography, well how do I explain this one? It means that…oh hell, I'll give it to you straight from *Mosby's Medical Dictionary*: "An array of detectors, positioned at several angles, records those x-rays that pass through the body." Now I am sure you feel fully informed after that definition. Let me try to simplify this, it is a machine that visually cuts the body in sections to better study what processes there may be going on inside. The area that is scanned will then print small pictures showing any abnormalities. This is great. In years past you would have surgery to do any exploring of the human body.

Since I had time to waste I figured that now was as good a

time as any to tell my head nurse I wouldn't be into work that day. My knees were still a little wobbly as I rode the elevator to the fifth floor of the hospital where I worked. I looked around and didn't see her so I asked the unit secretary if she was even around. She gave me a strange look and asked if I was all right. Was there something wrong? What's wrong, I thought, oh not much, George Bush (#1) was president and I had cancer, only two big problems that I could see. Too bad they were not both mistakes. She kept insisting I talk to her, but I knew that if I started I would not be able to control myself so I only shook my head.

I spotted one of the day nursing supervisors across the counter and asked if I could talk to her alone. We walked to the conference room behind the nurse's station. How many times I had seen physicians take families back there to deliver bad news. I guess it was my turn, now I was delivering the bad news. I told her that I wouldn't be in to work at least today because I had cancer. We hugged and cried. I told her that I was having a CT that afternoon and would hopefully know more later in the day when my doctor got the results back. After composing myself I left red faced, leaving her to tell everyone including my head nurse. I didn't want to talk about it. I just wanted it all to go away. Good old avoidance behavior, right?

How do you tell your mother that you have cancer, it isn't like telling her you have a cold, lost your car keys or are about to get married. I couldn't do it face to face so I took the coward's way out. I called her. I wasn't sure what to say as the phone to her office rang, when she answered I could barely say the words, "Mom, I have cancer."

She replied, "All right."

On the other side of the phone I didn't know what she was doing. I found out later she was trying not to choke on the words herself. She was trying to not let go and lose yet another of her children. I knew that she was in shock. Not much else was said after that, what really was there left to say? It has always been a joke between my mother and I that you deliver the bad news and

29

then she always responded with, "let me think about it and I'll call you back in two weeks."

Anyway that had been our usual running joke. Today it wasn't funny, and she never mentioned thinking about it.

An example of this, the time I called to tell her I was joining the Navy. After I told her she simply told me, "I have to think about it and I'll call you back in two weeks." You see she had to grant me permission as I was under the age of twenty-one. At that time any women needed parental consent if she was a minor. Men, on the other hand, could enter at seventeen without consent. But then again women were not on the front line as they are now. That is what equal rights have gotten us, being able to really get down in the trenches. I wonder if they still need parental consent, don't you?

When we arrived home, Jeff sat on the couch in our family room flipping through the channels, you know "channel-surfing." Something most men seem to do well. He wasn't really watching anything he was just flipping through and stopping for only a second. I, on the other hand, walked around the house smoking like a chimney. (Yes I was a smoker, and you noticed that it is past tense.) I paced back and forth. I simply couldn't sit still.

Later in the afternoon I started drinking and gagging on the CT contrast. Boy, I never thought anything of sending patients to x-ray for a CT scan before. I can remember telling the older patients, the ones in their seventies and eighties, you must drink this contrast or they cannot complete the test the doctor ordered. Sometimes we should all have to experience the things our patients do, it humbles you. Remember the movie *The Doctor*? If you happen to be in the medical community and haven't seen it; then you should rent or buy it.

After finishing the last drop of contrast I needed for the CT, Jeff and I headed back to the hospital. By the time we got there the news about me had spread throughout the whole place like a wildfire. So I shouldn't have been surprised when a friend of mine (who worked in the radiology department) gave me a big hug, assuring me all would be okay. Boy did I want what she was smoking or the crystal ball she was using. She sounded so sure I almost believed her. I didn't realize then that she was actually giving me a small ray of hope to cling to. Looking back on it now, I should have thanked her.

Once in the scanner room I was told to lie on this hard, cold table that moves forward very slowly as it scans. The machine itself was very noisy. It takes pictures at tiny intervals while you lie there in silence. The only voice I could hear, was a prerecorded message telling you to breathe in and hold, then exhale. I don't know about you but I have a hard time breathing on command. I felt like I was panting in between or needing to leak a little air out before I was told to exhale. I was left with only my thoughts, trying hard not to think at all just staring at the ceiling, which had an outdoor picture for me to look at.

After the x-ray we met the doctor in the emergency department conference room. He had the results of the CT scan with him. It was negative; believe it or not the silly thing could not locate any tumor. He told us that the mammogram was also negative. What could it be? I thought we were supposed to know something by now. How can you fight a disease if you don't know what or where the disease is? I thought to myself it really must be a mistake. He told us that Rochester was where I needed to go next; that the Mayo Clinic is used to figuring puzzles like this one out. The Mayo Clinic, wow, this is the big time. This was where everyone from around the world came to find causes for their ailments. Now I would be counted as one of those numbers.

Jeff finally broke his silence and spoke up asking the doctor if it meant anything that the rash I had seemed to form clusters around my veins. He seemed surprised to hear that. Then he assured us it wasn't anything like "leukemia" or something like that, if that was what we were thinking. He would get in touch with a doctor he knew in Rochester to help get me into the clinic system as soon as possible. He would call us once again after the appointments had been made. With that he exited swiftly out the door and down the corridor. Leaving us a little dumbfounded at first.

Then I was elated; *they couldn't find a tumor so perhaps it wasn't anything serious.* I thought. Jeff looked pensive which always concerned me, even today. You see I look to him for direction as to what my next cue would be. If anything didn't excite him then I wouldn't get too excited and so on. But him just becoming quiet made me think that *perhaps I should be nervous.*

That evening things were as normal as they could be in our house, considering what the morning had brought. The doctor kept his promise and called. I would be heading to Rochester on Monday, February 13, 1989. My God I can't wait that long! I asked him for something that would calm my nerves; he had offered it that morning but I turned him down. Now I could use it. I really couldn't believe I had to wait any longer. I was given a prescription for Xanax to help me survive the next few days.

When the children come home; oh, my God the children! What do I tell them? Jeff handled the situation perfectly; he didn't tell them anything definite. That Mommy was sick and we would be going to the Mayo Clinic next week to find out what it was. Children are so accepting. After Dad's explanation they went off to play. Boy, did I want to go and play, to forget.

Chapter Three

I DIDN'T WANT MY CHILDREN TO go through what I had. I wanted so much more for them, to have a happy family life that I had always dreamt of and once had. I thank God that Jeff dealt with them. I was too afraid! For the first time in my life I was actually speechless. A lot of people I know don't believe I was ever speechless just ask them.

I didn't want to die; I didn't want to think of dying. I guess I thought if no one talked about it, maybe it would just go away. Isn't it funny how the mind works when faced with a crisis? It tries to protect you any way it can. I was acting just like someone else I recall that said; "*Fiddly-dee I can't think about this today, I will think about this tomorrow.*"

Our beautiful children! Jennifer, eleven, would now grow up faster than I would have liked her to. She would have to help around the house more than she did, and then there was the possibility of having to face death at a young age. Justin, our son, the baby, was only eight not much younger than I was when I learned that people you love do go away.

At the age of nine I was faced with the loss of my brother. He was killed in a biking accident, as I mentioned earlier. What does a nine-year-old understand about death? I had argued with him that morning. I didn't want him to go biking with my other brother. I wanted him to go with me to pick wild raspberries by the railroad near our home. So naturally I believed I was the reason he died. At the end of the same year this was followed by the death of my stepfather in a car accident (he was the only father I knew). This was culminated by a near fatal car accident that involved my mother. My brother and I were separated from her for almost a year. My mother, brother and myself have made it through it all. We were and are survivors!

The next few days seemed to crawl by. I didn't go to work. I reassured my head nurse that I would definitely be working my shift over the weekend though. I needed to work now. It would help keep my mind off of me, for a while. Besides, there were sick people to take care of that needed me. That was what I was trained to do, to care for those in need.

My favorite patient was still there, I thought she could cheer me up. I have cancer, the world needed to stop until I get this all figured out, doesn't it? At least that is what I thought. I have the power to slow it down, don't I? I didn't want to miss anything. I was the center of my universe, so if things were not going well with me then everything would just have to stand still until it could be made right. Life does go on though, the minutes tick by, people still go to work, children grow up and the world goes on spinning in its orbit even if I have cancer. I realize I didn't have any power; cancer was calling the shots now.

I had read someplace that laughter can help combat disease.

Humor can distract us from our painful thoughts as well as physical pain. For the moment, the effect brought on by a humorous thought is occupying our mind with something other than the thoughts that are painful for us to dwell on.

One example is the "tension headache." If you can change the mood or change the surroundings so the source of tension is removed it gives the headache a chance to dissolve. I always need to have the last laugh; usually I am found to be the joker in the group. (Mind you, I never did go the extreme and do the lampshade on the head thing.) Little did I know that my sense of humor would help me. Through my experience, I believe that we all could use more humor in our lives.

It has been reported that children laugh, I mean belly laugh as much as four hundred times a day. Adults laugh maybe fifteen times a day. I guess things aren't as funny the older we get. I think they ought to be.

It has been said that laughter has been proven to bolster the body's immune system; it activates T-cells in the immune system. These are antibodies that fight against harmful microorganisms. Besides reading the Bible every day, perhaps a comic book or two should also be prescribed. It is no longer just the apple a day that keeps the doctor away; Archie and Jughead comic books are good for your soul too. Archie and Jughead, boy does that date me! I guess today, it would be Spiderman, X-Men or some other cyber hero today.

There are several other benefits to humor; it can lighten up any situation. Have you ever been to a lecture or talk where the instructor or teacher falls off the platform? I have and believe me it was hilarious. But then again, I laugh when I fall UP the stairs! "Laughter gives seriousness a break," this is my motto now.

I have told nursing students when I have been invited to share my story with them, that there isn't anything anymore that I take seriously, except perhaps a Code Blue (which is a cardiac arrest at our hospital). It is true! I can often be heard telling the other staff members on the unit to "lighten up." Whenever our mood and thoughts lighten up, it helps to relax our physical body. Sometimes I even need reminding of this myself.

The other day I was ranting and raving about the inadequate staffing at our hospital and mid-sentence my head nurse looked over at me and told me to "Cool it!" It sure lightened up the situation. In fact, there was dead silence until we all cracked up.

There are healthcare professionals who would like to see laughter become part of every patient's prescription. Wouldn't you like to say "Give the patient two aspirin along with a double dose of laughter and call me in the morning?" If there was something that could strengthen the immune system, which is better than a pill costing $100 dollars or more, wouldn't you try it? I believe that's highway robbery with the rising cost of prescription drugs. Everyone needs something that could help and laughter is free with no side effects

Believe it or not there are a few universities that are taking research a step further by helping to develop a software program that will allow doctors to create customized laughter prescriptions. By asking patients what makes them laugh, doctors can then create an individualized humor report. My hope is that they can get this off the ground.

I have become a firm believer in complementary, alternative, and preventative medicine. Things like: massage, reflexology, YOGA, tai chi, music therapy, and the list is endless. They are other ways to help your body. Take care of yourself now with whatever resources are available and you could possibly avoid paying for it later and that isn't funny it's true.

Therapeutic humor is defined as: "any intervention that promotes health and wellness by stimulating a playful discovery, expression or appreciation of the absurdity or incongruity of life's situations. This intervention may enhance health or be used as a complementary treatment of illness to facilitate healing or coping, whether physical, emotion, cognitive, social, or spiritual."

You do know that some people when faced with a stressful situation will oftentimes laugh uncontrollably. I know at times I will, because if I didn't laugh I would cry. Laughter is the greatest healer known to man, *to Laugh* (in my opinion) *is to Love and to Love is to Live*. Here is a quote from one of my favorite old movies, *Auntie Mame*. Mame tells everyone that you need to "*Live, live, live! Life is a banquet and most poor suckers are starving to death.*" Every time I hear that I chuckle to myself. I want to have that attitude. I want to experience it all! I want to gorge myself on a big helping of love and life. I could expound on this further by quoting more researchers, theories or old movies, but I think that Mame said it all.

I went to work that Saturday trying to carry on as though nothing was wrong. I was after all my mother's daughter, strong, stoic, stiff upper lip you know (a good Brit). Let's keep up the pretense that nothing has changed, you can crumble only on the inside. Remember to smile and wave when joining in the parade. My life will go on as normal, right? I learned my lessons well. I also believe that in my life this is much of the reason I have come this far. Not being drowned by the moment or situation, just pick myself up by the bootstraps and press on.

No one at work would leave me alone. They were all eager to tell me how sorry they were. Asking for all the details, some even wanted to see the rash. I felt I was now the hospital sideshow. I felt that I couldn't handle taking care of my favorite patient. I didn't want to get into it with her, she had enough on her own plate to deal with in her life, and she didn't need to fret over me. I regret not sharing that particular part of my life with her; she may have been able to take care of me a little; after all, we were friends. Isn't that what friends do, take care of each other?

I asked to not be assigned to her avoiding her and her room totally. By the weekend she was wondering why I hadn't come in to see her. It had been reported to me that she was getting weaker. The doctors were not sure how long she had to live. I have often wondered if she didn't know that something was very wrong with me. I think about whether or not she sensed I too was sick. I don't know if I will ever understand how we as humans, who have been given the gift of speech, never have learned to tell someone how we really feel. The young and the old are the only ones that *tell it like it is*. They have no inhibitions; they are not caught up in the mumble-jumble that we in the middle years seem to have. At the end of the weekend I finally found enough courage to go in and see her.

I bounced through the door in my usual manner. I wasn't prepared to see what I saw. She was just a shell of the girl I had known for these past few months, so frail and pale. I apologized for not coming by sooner and proceeded to give her some lame excuse that the patients I was caring for were far more needy than

37

I thought they would be. I could see she wasn't really buying it, yet I continued on with the facade. I was another Sara Bernhardt in the making. I could fool the best of them, couldn't I? Or is it only in the dark. Did I really fool her or was she allowing me to deal with it on my own?

I walked around her room. Only the dim light from the bathroom and the hallway by the nurse's station shone in on us. I paced around the small room looking at pictures on the wall. They were ones I had seen a thousand times before. I found myself daydreaming only hearing her small voice in the background speaking quietly. I didn't really hear what she was saying. I was there in body only. I was gone in spirit.

She was a Gary Larson fan; the author of the *Far Side*, everything in her room was decorated with some kind of *Far Side* paraphernalia. Oh how happy she was the day he called her from his home in Seattle.

One day her doctor told us that she would not live to get out of the hospital and that if anyone could contact the Make A Wish Foundation or something like that to please do it. She was too old for help from the Make a Wish Foundation, they had an age limit and it was eighteen, she was twenty-six. I took this as a personal challenge. The next morning I made many phone calls telling my story until someone finally listened to me. It was at Gary Larson's publishing company that I was able to hook up to him. This woman I talked with told me she could call Gary and if he were in the United States she would see if he could call my patient. He called the same day. They talked for almost an hour, it was so good to see her laugh and be happy. The hospital had made arrangements with the person that ran the photography department to video their conversation for her family.

Oh, my dear friend, I am so sorry I never was strong enough to talk to you about what was happening to me. You see I was taught long ago that you hide your pain, sorrow and fears inside. I am apologizing for not being there when you died to just say good-bye. Yet maybe that night in the dark we did say our good-byes. Even then I was the weak one. I couldn't face your death;

I couldn't face the possibility that I could die too.

On Friday I gathered my x-rays, lab reports, and even that damn pathology report from the different clinics. On the way out of the building I ran into one of the oncology doctors at our hospital, he gave me a big hug. He also told me to go to Rochester, they would find out what it was, and then I could come home and be treated. It wasn't that the hospital I worked at wasn't capable of finding out what I was dealing with, it's that compared in size to our facility the Mayo Clinic was like comparing David to Goliath. We were just too small.

Our lab on a daily basis may handle 50 outpatients. The Mayo Clinic handles thousands. So along with the convenience of the clinic being only one and a half hours away it made sense for me to go there to find a diagnosis. You realize this was before the time of HMOs, PPOs and any other kind of "O" they can find to throw at us that dictate medical treatment. Waiting for approval from an insurance company to make decisions on treatment courses or which medications are approved to prescribe could actually kill any of us. For instance, doctors often submit the correct forms on a leukemia patient, but cannot start treatment until they receive permission. Someone's life may be hanging in the balance and they have think about it? What's wrong with that picture?

When Monday finally came Jeff and I woke up at four-thirty in the morning. We needed to arrive at the clinic by seven. I remember taking my shower in tears, I discovered as time went on that the shower was always a good place for me to release my real feelings. No one could hear me sobbing or crying above the sound of the water beating on the fiberglass walls. As for my red face, if someone asked why I simply blamed it on the hot water. The shower was often my refuge many more times through the years. We dressed in silence both afraid of what the day might bring. We seemed dazed by what was happening, kind of like when you catch a deer in your headlights. It's as if your feet were buried in cement.

I glanced down at my chest, now peppered with the stupid red bumps. They both disgusted and scared the hell out of me at the same time. In the morning when I woke I would pull my nightgown away from my skin to see if by chance sleep made them simply disappear. No such luck! They were always there glaring back at me, letting me know that this cancer thing was in control, not me. This was very hard for me since I am a well-known control freak. Just ask my family!

My mother was in the kitchen when I walked in; she was making coffee, remember she was living with us. I just stood there while she put her arms around me, I couldn't bring myself to return the gesture, and I was still too numb. She seemed to be trying to comfort both of us.

My mother was always the strong one in the family. Through all of our family tragedies I remember her being as steady as a rock. Do you suppose she too found solace in her shower time as I did? She had suffered so many things in her life. One way to deal with a tragedy is to put it at arm's length while you process all information, sound familiar? Not this morning though, the morning I was going to Rochester, she cried. She always told me you never get over the death of a child. I wondered, was she remembering my brother as she held on to me that early morning.

What would she do if she lost two children? Having never experienced the loss of a child as a mother I could only imagine what she was feeling. My mother has only mentioned briefly always with emotion in her voice that the loss of a child is like no other loss you could experience. The pain is indescribable. I know that is why every time the year rolls around to April, the month of my brother's birth or the month of July, the month of his death, these are extremely hard dates for her, as is for all of us. God bless you, Mom! I promise that I will survive. You taught me how.

The children came downstairs to see us off; this broke the silence of the moment. I don't believe anyone slept well the night before, except the children. They weren't aware of the crisis our family was facing. I had my medication. It was the only way I could face the long nights now, so my sleep was like being in a coma.

I now understand why patients are so restless at night, because the nights are dark, scary, and very long. The children simply had their innocence, all they knew was that Mom was sick. From the vast knowledge of life at their ages I'm sure they couldn't understand why they just didn't give me Tylenol, tell me to gargle with salt water, or put a Band-Aid on it. There would be no Band-Aid this time kiddies, this was definitely bigger than anything Johnson & Johnson could make. This boo-boo was larger than any they had seen. It was hard to make them understand what was happening to our home life. Especially when we couldn't make sense of it ourselves.

Chapter Four

THE DRIVE TO ROCHESTER WAS A long one. The sound of the tires as they clickity-clacked down the highway at times was deafening. I didn't realize that when the material they used to pave the highway changed so did the noises the tires made. It had snowed the night before so this added to the variety of the sounds of the road as we moved along.

Have you ever noticed that after our winters in the north, the roads become even bumpier? I suppose the road crews wouldn't have much to do if they didn't have repairs to fix after the winter. Jeff says that it has something to do with the expanding and contracting of the pavement from all the ice and snow packed down on them during the winter months. I guess it made sense. At least I've not heard of anything to the contrary.

It started spitting snow as we traveled along. I watched as occasionally a snowflake would land on the windshield then melt or get swept away by the cadence of the wipers. Snowflakes are enchanting. No two are alike, that is the thing that amazes me the most. If you are lucky enough to find a large one sometimes you will even be able to make out its design. I wished my troubles could melt or be swept away by the wipers as easy as the snowflakes.

Jeff and I remained still, sitting up straight in our seats, staring off in the darkness of the early morning. The headlights from oncoming cars seemed to cut through the endless darkness like a knife. I wanted desperately to talk to him, to try and comfort him, or have him comfort me. I didn't know how or what to say. The words didn't come to either of us, just the damn silence. Normally a drive like this wouldn't be a problem, because when we travel somewhere I would fall asleep almost before we left the driveway. Not on this day. I couldn't sleep. We were both so quiet we could hear the other breathing.

The minutes ticked by at a slow pace. You could now see off in the distance the sky on the horizon was starting to lighten up. It was as if a blanket was being lifted, unfolding and bringing hope to a new day. The sun coming up was especially beautiful that morning, or was it that I was being more attentive to my surroundings. The brighter it got the more the snow on the ground glistened.

How looks can be deceiving, I thought. It was actually bitterly cold out there. The car being warmed by the sun found me wanting to curl up in a ball and take a nap, just like a kitten. I would catch myself dozing off from time to time dreaming momentarily of happier times before the rash, only to be jolted back to reality when the car hit a rut in the road.

I can't tell you the feeling I had as we came over the hill that led into Rochester. It was like going up and down on a roller coaster, shouting, "I had just lost my stomach." Up ahead there they stood tall, gray, and cold, the Mayo Clinic buildings. I never knew how big they really were. It was awesome, even though the sight sickened me all at the same time. I could feel my heart race, as the rush of adrenaline came over me once again. Fear! Let's tell it like it is…I was damn scared!

This time there wasn't a choice. I couldn't run away. I would have to take a stand and fight. I would beat this giant! Just like David beat Goliath, with a sense of hope and faith it would be conquered. CANCER. I decided I would not lose my husband, children or the life that we had created. I reached over and touched Jeff's hand briefly. He closed his hand around mine and gave it a squeeze as he continued to look straight ahead. My hands were like ice cubes and the warmth I felt from his comforted me. I could feel my heart pound so hard it was as if it were going to jump out of my chest. I sighed heavily as we pulled into the parking ramp. I know now that this was the beginning of my panic attacks; something I would continue to be plagued with over the years.

After parking the car we made our way to a small clinic doorway. It was dwarfed in size compared to the skyscrapers making up the other Mayo Clinic buildings. It wasn't attached to the other buildings. It sort of stood off by itself. That alone made it not as overwhelming as the old dinosaurs that loomed overhead.

We scurried inside to the reception desk; just like white lab rats trying to find their way through a maze. Only we were simply trying to get in out of the cold. The receptionist confirmed that they were expecting me but not until nine. Surprise we were two hours early. They apologized for the misunderstanding, but they wouldn't be open for business until normal clinic hours that started at nine o'clock. I glanced at my watch. Wow, it was only seven. My husband would never believe I was early to anything, let alone two hours early, if he hadn't been there to see it for himself. History has often proven that I rarely am early for things. I am either on time or late, but never early.

The receptionist said, "I am going to send you to the lab to have some more blood drawn. You also need to give us a urine sample. Then you can have breakfast, just plan to be back by nine of course." We nodded and exited through the nearest door.

Oh great I thought, what a way to start off, arriving too early. It is the waiting that gets to me the most. I can remember a saying we had when I was in the Navy, "*hurry up and wait.*" No matter what it was you always ended up waiting for someone or something. I discovered later on that this is true not just to the military but also in all walks of life.

44

I have never been one for patience. You could say it isn't a virtue of mine. I'm one of those people who blows her horn in traffic jams, who switches checkout lanes if I think I can get through somewhere else faster. So telling me to wait until nine was like putting me in the wrong checkout lane. All I could think about was how we could have slept longer. We could have left home in the daylight instead of what seemed to be the middle of the night. Although, I think that if we had left later in the morning we would have missed the beauty we encountered on our drive.

I have read somewhere that patience is the art of waiting, taking time to master. I have already told you that I have little to no patience being honest with you. So, mastering any part of it sounds unfamiliar. How does one do that? Having one's patience tried more often? Perhaps that is why I am chronically late for things. Try to think of it this way; at least I don't have to wait as long.

We left the clinic and started out in search of a local McDonald's because it was cheap and fast. They had many little restaurants near the clinic but no McDonald's. We finally found one two miles away. Jeff ordered his usual Egg McMuffin, a large orange juice and coffee. I wasn't hungry so I ordered a large orange juice. The smell of his breakfast was tempting but I was afraid to eat. I was too nauseated. I guess through the power of suggestion I could feel myself actually becoming sick. I was told so many times I was ill, that I was now starting to play the role. The power of the mind, a small drop of information, "I'm sick! I am sorry to hear you're sick. I hope you get better soon." Then presto, you are sick!

We arrived back at the clinic, at precisely nine o'clock. Not long after we arrived, we were led into an exam room where I was handed a gown to change into. It wasn't until I was in the dressing room that I noticed there were no armholes in the gown. I didn't know which way to put it on. I was chuckling to myself behind the drawn curtain; I thought this had to be some kind of a joke. I was looking around to see if someone was going to pop up and yell, "Smile, you're on *Candid Camera*."

45

That would have been great for a little comic relief. Naturally, being the dutiful patient I tied the gown in front like a Superman cape. Stepping from the change room the doctor politely turned it around for me so as to no longer expose my breasts. I was so embarrassed thinking *here I am a college graduate* and I can't even put a gown on the right way. It didn't seem to bother him, he never missed a beat, he continued with his explanation of how I would be "dumped" into the Mayo Clinic system by seeing him first. After that I was going to be referred to an oncologist. Evidently it takes months to get into the clinic unless you have some kind connection. It's a way to cut through the red tape. I was glad that we did it this way. I couldn't imagine waiting months for a diagnosis. Even if I was learning patience, that would be asking too much even of a patient person.

I had a thorough going-over by this doctor. Examining me from head to toe then back again. I even had another pap smear, breast exam, and if he had his way he would like to have done another skin biopsy. Boy, what good was it to get started back home, when they repeated everything up here? He finally decided to hold off on the biopsy. He told us he'd wait until after I went to the Oncology Department. "They may want to do this themselves," he said. It was a relief, because if he wanted to biopsy this, and then they wanted to biopsy it where would that leave me? On the other hand, maybe they could simply biopsy them all off then I wouldn't have cancer.

We thanked him and left with a small folder that held a map along with other little folders. These told me the different areas of the clinic I needed to report to. He patted me on the back, shook my husband's hand wishing us good luck. I didn't even get a lollipop for being a good patient! I would never see him again; in fact, even though I swore I wouldn't, I've even forgotten his name.

First, we were off to the clinic laboratory department. We walked down this ramp that entered into a corridor where hundreds of people at various speeds went whipping passed us. You better go with the flow and not stop or people doing the

46

hundred-yard dash while talking on cell phones could easily run you down. Women/men of all nationalities, shapes and sizes in business or jogging suits wearing sneakers heading somewhere. Some limped, others used crutches, and still others were being pushed in wheelchairs. It was amazing!

We got lost a few times that first day while wandering around trying to follow the little maps. It's funny to think back on it. We now know the clinic system along with the buildings like the back of our hands. It doesn't even look like an unfriendly giant as it once did. It reminded me of hearing of another time in history when all the sick people gathered to be healed by one man. Now they come to the Mayo Clinic, brought to you by the brothers Mayo.

I am a people watcher by nature; I could sit in an airport, on a bench in a park, or just stroll the mall somewhere and watch people go by. I often wonder what is going on in their lives and what has brought them here? Are they happy or sad, relaxed, stressed, befuddled, lost or just as scared as we were? During all this time we spent together that day, we continued to do it in utter silence. Still too afraid to speak. Yet we did touch, holding hands, a pat on the back or an arm around the other. Simple gestures that spoke volumes to me, making me feel that I was not alone in all of this.

Chapter Five

THE LABORATORY DEPARTMENT WAS LIKE NONE I had ever seen. It consisted of a large desk in a half moon shape. Behind it sat several women dressed in white, punching lab folders into a time clock while asking people when was their last meal. I explained that we were from another clinic and that I had already had my blood drawn. She raised her eyebrow peering over her half rimmed glasses uttering merely, "Oh."

Since then I too have worn those little half glasses, and I too found myself peering over the rims the same way she did. Seeing her do the same made me chuckle. I do believe wearing the little things is a sign of getting older. I say it is only my way of being age fashionable. Mine were speckled with all the primary colors; my daughter says they suited me well. I have since had cataract surgery on both eyes and no longer need the half glasses. But as the time goes on I am contemplating going back to them, just because they're cute.

She looked me up one side and down the other. With some disdain she slipped away to another part of the desk. There she picked up the phone dialing a number and glancing back at me momentarily. She swiftly turned around so I couldn't hear what she was saying. I couldn't imagine what I had done to her other than interrupt her little well rehearsed speech.

A few moments later she returned bringing with her the same stern expression. Again peering over her glasses, she explained these were additional lab tests I needed to have done. This time she was a little too smug. With a tight-lipped smile on her face as she handed me back the remainder of my clinic folders. As she shoved the folder at me she directed me to the colored chairs where I was to wait for my name to be called.

We walked around the desk behind her just as she directed, as I looked back she was whispering to one of the other ladies working with her at the desk pointing to me. I simply smiled and nodded back at her. I thought to myself, *what a bitch*. I wanted to stick my tongue out at her. I wonder what she would have done then. Instead I decided to mind my "p"s and "q"s, which pleased Jeff immensely.

Sure enough there were color coded chairs in long rows, orange, blue, yellow and purple, there had to be at least one hundred plus of them. In front of the pack were matching colored doors. Obediently we took our seats and waited for my name to be called. Finally, along with at least eight other people it was my turn. I was to report to the blue section. A different lady in white with a nasally sounding voice was calling me. The colored doors reminded me of the old TV show *Let's Make a Deal*. *What's behind door number one?* I thought to myself. Or in my case what was behind the blue door? I would have been a lot happier if it had been a new car. I was surprised to simply find another small room, smaller than the one I had just been in. It was at this point that Jeff and I were briefly separated, which made me a bit nervous because I needed him now. I took a chair and one more time waited to hear my name called from behind a small curtain. Boy, what a system!

When I heard my name I followed what I figured to be a lab technician, a phlebotomist to be exact. She asked me to roll up my sleeve past my elbow. After repeating my name and spelling it for her, I wondered if she honestly thought someone else would come in here and have their blood drawn if they didn't have to. Not me, I hated needles and made no qualms about telling anyone either. Unfortunately for me I have the world's worst veins (I know that's what they all say), and they were destined to become much worse. Only recently I found out it must be a hereditary trait to some degree. My mother and at least one of her sisters have very poor veins too.

The phlebotomist carried with her a small tray of blood sample tubes. All of them had colored tops and labels attached to them, with my name and identification number that I had been assigned earlier that morning. I told her that the left arm would probably be her best bet. She nodded and began searching my arm. She found her target quickly.

When the last bit of blood was drawn she covered the area with a gauze sponge, and then wrapped it with a small roll of gauze tucking the end inside. I was instructed to leave this on for at least fifteen minutes. After that she turned away to put my blood samples in a small conveyor for processing. Smiling she politely said, "Have a good day." Right, I thought how could I have a good day with what the results might hold from the blood she drew. How impersonal they were here, numbers, names and little colored chairs with matching doors.

I collected Jeff from the waiting room and headed for the Mayo building itself where we took the elevator getting off on the twelfth floor. This was the Oncology floor; we were to report to twelve east to be exact. We were in for our next shock of the day, there are over fifty oncologists at the Mayo Clinic, believe me I counted. Not much else to do while we waited. We went to the reception desk and asked about our appointment, handing the receptionist my little white clinic folder.

She told us, "I don't have an opening for today. But we can set up for you to have an appointment for tomorrow." Oh, my God, we would have to return the next day! The thought of coming back for another day made me nauseous all over again.

My cancer diagnosis was just as out of reach as trying to catch the "elusive" butterfly. That's the way I felt at that moment. Jeff and I took only a minute to discuss it. We decided that as tired as we were, even though we really wanted to know something. It would probably be smarter to come back in the morning when we would actually have an appointment. We told her we would happily take the one-thirty afternoon appointment she had for the next day. We turned to leave rushing toward the elevator.

It was mid-afternoon; around two o'clock when we started our long drive home. Again traveling the distance in silence. We were each deep in our own thoughts. Exhausted from the strain of the morning and not finding anything out, add to this getting up early was all quite a test of our patience. I dozed off and on, being almost once again hypnotized by the clickity-clack of the road noises.

Suddenly, I startled myself awake. My thoughts instantly ran back to my favorite patient at the hospital. For some odd reason I was feeling a deep sense of loss, like being alone. When we arrived home I found out that she passed away that afternoon at about two-thirty, which was about the time I suddenly awoke from my nap. She was far too young. Yet she would no longer be in pain, I thought. Why do we always say that when someone dies? Would someone think that of me when I was gone? I forced myself to stop thinking that way. I was not going to die! I would beat cancer! I would not have it beat me!

It was awhile after her death, when I was a patient myself that I received a letter from her mother telling me that I now had a new angel to watch over me…After reading that I sat on the edge of my hospital bed dropping the envelope and watched as it slid to the floor in slow motion. There I sat looking out the window while a tear slowly slid down my cheek. I still miss her today, when I think of her my eyes will still well up with tears.

Once home we received a lot of phone calls that night. Everyone wanted to know what we had found out, what was the diagnosis. Jeff fielded all the calls. I didn't want to talk to anyone. I took my Xanax and zoned out in front of the TV for a while, only toying with slumber. I was tired and not very happy that we came back empty-handed. My patience was really being tried, could this mean I was mastering patience. I was told once that if you pray for patience that you would only be tested more to teach you how to become patient. If that is true, then is the reverse of this also true? If you pray to be tested more will patience automatically be given to you? This is something to think about!

Later that evening a close family friend visited us. She and I worked together before I got into school to get my nursing degree! We had both worked as admitting clerks in the Emergency Department part-time. She worked to keep from getting bored. I worked so I could get my foot in the door at the hospital in a time when there was not a nursing shortage.

It was probably lucky that she had her job in the department because when she and her husband separated; she was able to continue on there and not have to start looking for a job to support herself. She was older than most of the other part-time admitting clerks and seeing as I was no spring chicken myself we hit it off well. We always worked good together sharing a lot of laughs, even on the job. This was the beginning of realizing how much laughter helps. It gives a cathartic like release, but do remember that the key word is appropriate laughter; we all know the right and wrong time to cut up.

Coincidentally, when I graduated from nurses training she took a full-time job in the front admitting office. She had flexible hours with every other Wednesday, Thursday and Friday off. It was great so we usually planned little road trips. That night she stopped over to see what we had heard from the trip to Mayo. We told her that we knew nothing more than we already knew and that when we did we'd let her know. She stayed awhile longer after that, the visit was somewhat strained by everyone's thoughts of the next day's trip. We were all searching for answers and no one wanted one more than me. Yet we were all afraid of what we might find out.

My aunt, my mother's youngest sister, was also going to Rochester trying to find a diagnosis for a memory loss problem she was having. She called that night too, during the conversation we decided that the next day we would all travel up to Mayo together.

In the early morning we headed north one more time we hoped. We took the back roads instead of the interstate. Not as many cars on the road this route so it seemed even more like the middle of night. This time the car wasn't as somber, as it had been the day before. In fact, we laughed and joked most of the way. My aunt kept the conversation rolling along telling her jokes about the fact she thought she was losing her memory/mind. It certainly helped keep our minds off what was going on in our own lives. It always helps to listen to someone else's problems because it takes the focus off you.

When we arrived I needed to give more blood samples (the vampires), my aunt needed to have her head CT scan repeated. Naturally they wanted to repeat the one she had done at home. Over the years I found that the doctors simply like to have things done in their own facility (that is changing now because of the rising cost of health insurance coverage). Having people they know read the results. I sometimes think that Mayo believes that we have our vets and doctors practicing together in Iowa. We pay for our services on the barter system. A chicken for a checkup, perhaps a dozen eggs for cold medicine. Well this is not true, we have most of the same equipment they have, just on a much smaller scale.

Back to the desk in the lab with the not so nice lady dressed in white. This time I wanted even more to stick my tongue out at her but Jeff said I couldn't. I simply smiled politely gritting my teeth the whole time.

After we were done in the lab, we were off to 3-East, Radiology. I needed a chest x-ray, believe it or not, I never had one all this time. This is where for a while we were separated from my aunt. It took her longer for her CT scan than it did for my chest x-ray. Jeff and I decided we would go to the cafeteria while we waited for her. We told her we would return in about an hour to collect her. The day was actually going well and I was feeling guilty for not being more depressed.

When we finally met up with her again, we only had a few moments before my doctor's appointment. Next she needed to go to the eighth floor to see her doctor and we made our way back to the twelfth floor Oncology Clinic.

While sitting in the waiting room we listened again for my name to be called. People sat there discussing their cancers as if they were talking about a common cold. They were laughing and joking, discussing who had or had not been cured. Sharing side effects of treatment, what helped and what didn't. Jeff and I were truly amazed by this; we weren't expecting this kind of laissez-faire attitude. We thought that when you have cancer that you all just sit and quietly wait your fate. Eventually you died.

My impression of what people with cancer were like was completely out of line; at least that is what I was discovering. People who have cancer are a special breed. They seem to have found the meaning of life. Whatever time that they were left with, albeit one day, one week, one year or perhaps only one more hour they would make the most of that time. Are you starting to get a glimpse of what I am talking about when I said to have cancer is a "privilege." It is like being blind and still being able to see. These people here in the waiting room were just that "privileged."

At the time we didn't know this so we sat in awe of what we both were hearing. It somehow made us feel hopeful; even if I had cancer it could be fixable. Looking at all these people who were not only being treated but were learning how to live with their cancers not die from them. It goes to the drinking glass theory. Is the glass half empty or is it half full? Would I live my remaining years down and out, or would I live my life free and happy? These were the questions I was now asking myself instead of looking in the yellow pages for a funeral home or lawyer to make out my will. I was going to live, by God! Live!

I had become hypnotized just listening to these wonderful people. Finally, I heard from somewhere off in the distance, my name being called. My heart started pounding, whoever said the only thing to fear is fear itself must not have had to face cancer or any other life-threatening circumstance. We pitifully followed the nurse down the hall to one of the exam rooms.

Nothing fancy, just the familiar exam table, dressing room and a desk with a computer on it. There was also a long couch instead of chairs where we both sat waiting for our next instructions. I kept heaving those heavy sighs that always came whenever I was overly stressed. This was like fingernails running down a chalkboard from the way Jeff reacted each time I did this. He finally told me to stop. *He speaks*, I thought, he hadn't said more than a few words to me in days. It was nice to hear he still had his voice, even if he used it to chastise me.

Jeff was raised in a "normal" family, not really facing much adversity while he was growing up. I didn't know if he knew how to handle such things. Though, he seemed to be holding up quite well under the pressure. Looking back now I think he was like a simmering pot sitting on a back burner, waiting to blow its lid off. He apologized for yelling and said it was because he was nervous, I thought to myself, *That's why I sigh.*

Just then the door swung open to see a very nice looking man in his mid-forties with sandy brown hair and blue eyes. When he spoke I immediately was mesmerized, he had a British accent. Being from the generation that grew up with The Beatles, Herman's Hermits, and the Rolling Stones made me love British accents. I must have looked like a complete idiot with my mouth hanging open, because he asked me if I was okay. *Okay*, I thought, now I am totally embarrassed. I managed to tell him I was fine.

He had reviewed my "portfolio"; I assumed he meant my chart. He couldn't actually give me a complete diagnosis at that time. My God, no! Not after all the blood work they had done and the x-rays that were shot, how could he not have something to tell me! He continued by saying that he could tell us that it wasn't a tumor. My blood work along with the other tests had ruled that out. He now believed we were dealing with a hematological (blood) problem and unfortunately that was out of his level of expertise. How could he tell me that out of the many oncologists I had met one who couldn't give me a diagnosis; that was out of his range of expertise? I was getting edgy and he could sense it.

To get a more conclusive picture, he needed to perform another test...a bone marrow aspirate and biopsy. I wanted to faint! Oh, no, not that! You can have all the blood I have but to say I needed a bone marrow biopsy scared the hell out of me. I was scheduled for one that afternoon to be taken from both hips. He would have the results tomorrow, at which time he would have a hematologist join us. He would be better able to explain the results and the course of treatment at that time.

Looking at the doctor, Jeff asked, "Don't you have an idea as to what we are being faced with?" Me, I couldn't say anything, I was horrified. I was trying not to let my stomach or heart jump out of my chest. I have to have a bone marrow. I kept thinking, *Calm down, Jeanine, just because you assisted with them in the Navy doesn't mean they still do it the same way.* Look at how far medicine has advanced in nearly twenty years. Maybe it's a simpler procedure now! *Yes,* I thought, *he was right, it wouldn't be as bad as I remembered...would it?*

I sensed the doctor could see that after our many days of exhausting rounds made from clinic to clinic, lab to lab, we were close to the end of our rope. Before exiting the room he turned and said he thought it was possibly a type of "lymphoma." With that he shook our hands and left. Lymphoma, that we can live with, no one dies from that anymore!

Jeff seemed almost elated with that news; he made it easy to get caught up in his enthusiasm too! It was as if he'd been awakened from a long nap or gotten his second wind. When the oncologist left the room and the door swung closed it blew life back into us again! Okay, Rip Van Winkle, thank God it didn't take us forty years to wake up. Before heading home we gathered all the pamphlets we could find in the waiting room about lymphoma. We wanted to be well informed for the next day's meeting with the hematologist.

Chapter Six

WE LEFT THE TWELFTH FLOOR, HEADING back to the Hilton Building and down into the subway, where outpatient bone marrow biopsies were performed. It was behind the lab section where we had started earlier that morning; an area I refer to as the torture chamber. I checked in and sat in the small waiting room while Jeff went off in search of my aunt. We didn't know where she had vanished to; besides, if she was truly having memory problems we could only imagine where she may have wandered off. I told him to hurry back because I didn't want to go through this thing alone. I kept looking down the corridor to see if he was heading back in my direction, no such luck, he disappeared into the crowd. "Coward," I mumbled under my breath!

I sat there for about fifteen minutes when I heard my name called. Wouldn't you figure I wasn't going to wait an hour or two for this like I did everything else? I could get in right away. I glanced around the waiting room; I was the only one there. I guess they don't have people beating down the doors for a bone marrow biopsy. No colored chairs with matching doors, no other waiting rooms. This was it and they were ready for me, I looked once again, still no Jeff in sight. I sighed, slowly getting to my feet on legs made of Jell-O and walked to the open door. I did take one more glance back before the door closed in case Jeff had suddenly reappeared. No such luck!

A young man led me down the hall to another small room where I was about to experience the worst pain of my life. I asked the lady, if she would give me something to knock me out, she laughed and said that even though she would like to they didn't pre-medicate anyone for this procedure. That the next time I should get something ordered from my doctor. What, was she crazy! I wasn't going to have any more of these. All I could do now was bite the bullet; I thought, *If you hurt me I'm simply going to hurt you back.* My heart was in my throat and my stomach kept doing flip-flops. If these were butterflies they must have been the size of robins. I couldn't make up my mind if I needed to throw up or just pass out.

She explained the procedure telling me she too was an RN and had been trained to do this procedure. I asked her if she had done very many before, trying to make small talk not questioning her. I didn't want her to get the impression that I was checking her competency. I just wanted to stall the inevitable event for a while, for as long as I could. I smiled and followed her instructions. I was to lie on my stomach on the table, and undo the jeans I was wearing to expose my backside. A bone marrow biopsy is drawn from the back of the hips, technically called the iliac crest, a flat bone in the rump area.

"I'll explain everything as we go along, okay?" she asked. I nodded, I was so frightened I couldn't move or speak! "I'm going to cover you with a drape and pull your jeans down a little lower. Now, I'm just going to press down on the bone to find my landmarks." With each sentence she always added that "now." She worked swiftly, with precision and she seemed quite knowledgeable even though her instructions were like all the other well-rehearsed speeches I had been hearing over the last two days.

"Now I'm going to give you some lidocaine to numb the area, it will feel like a rubber band snap," she said, and it did.

"Ouch!" I complained.

"I'm sorry, but I did tell you that it would feel like a rubber band snap," she remarked. She continued talking and explaining the entire procedure. All I thought of was it had to be one hell of a rubber band!

I know that they must have put me in a soundproof room because; while I was sitting in the waiting room I never heard a sound coming from inside. I realized, that the sounds I was making while she jabbed me must have sounded like a cow delivering a calf. She kept telling me to breathe because I would hold my breath from time to time. Finally, I found panting like they teach in Lamaze classes was a good way to get some needed oxygen to my brain and stay focused.

She finally pulled the long needle from my backside, covered the area with a big bulky pressure dressing and told me that she would let me have a five-minute break before doing the other side. I started crying. I couldn't believe that I was going to have to do it again. Where was my rat of a husband? He deserted me, just like a rat leaving a sinking ship. I sobbed and tried not to let them know I was a big baby.

"It's really okay to cry, honey," she said very gently. "I know it hurts, and we will get the next one done as fast as we can." I am surprised she didn't start that with "now, honey." She did go fast or so it seemed. Or maybe it seemed fast because, whenever you go some place you have never been, it always take forever. But, on the return trip it seems to go much faster. Again, I held my breath, again I panted and again I uttered horrible sounds. After the final piece of tape was applied I was handed an instruction pamphlet explaining how to care for my bone marrow site, along with two band-aids. *They could have made them Snoopy Band-Aids*, I thought.

"Have a good day!" Those were her final words to me as she patted my shoulder. If I heard one more person tell me to have a good day I thought I would scream. They say it like we are on a Love Boat cruise, heading into port for a day of shopping. The purser yells, as you depart the ship "Have a good day!"

I hobbled down the hall to the waiting room where I was hoping to find Jeff, but no such luck. I couldn't imagine where he could be. Now that it was over, I felt I had to have been in there for hours. Imagine my surprise to see it had only been a half-hour. All that pain in only thirty minutes, this is better service than a lot of fast food places. And they smile and say, "have a good day" as well.

I finally found Jeff in front of the lab check-in desk, where the crabby lady I didn't like sat. I put my arms around him managing only a whisper, "They hurt me!" It was then that the floodgates opened, the pain was gone momentarily in my hips. I believe I was now crying over the stress of the past few days. I was crying like I did as a child, after I fell off of my bike skinning my knee. Yes, I was hurt but it seemed to hurt worse the closer I got to home. By the time I arrived, my mother thought I had cut off a limb. I didn't do brave well then when I was hurt, so I wasn't doing brave well now.

We headed back to the x-ray floor to find my aunt, who also listened to my tale of how much they had hurt me. She hugged me and said we should all go out for lunch that we deserved it. We went to the Red Lobster that was just down the street, where we shared both a good meal and good conversation. The trials and tribulations of the day seemed to melt away with the cheesecake I had for dessert.

We continued to talk all the way home just like we did on the way up. We went over the pamphlets Jeff had picked up on lymphoma, none of it sounded too bad. Yes, I would have to have chemotherapy. Yes, I would have to lose my hair and be sick but I wouldn't die. The survival rate was really quite good. We all felt very reassured by what the oncologist suspected.

When we arrived home my mother came out to the car to greet us followed by our children. They could hardly wait to hear the news. When we told them the suspicions held by the doctor, they couldn't help getting caught up in the excitement of the news too. I called my head nurse to give her the good news also. I felt that a big brick was lifted off my shoulders; I had been emotionally and physically spent. I had been rejuvenated some and even managed to cook dinner that evening. Once the dishes were done, I was able to spend quality time with my family.

While Jeff explained the ordeal to the children, my mother and I went to the hairdresser where she had made an appointment for me to have my hair washed. I was so weak and sick by then; remember I had cancer now so mentally I became sick. She thought I would feel better if I had someone wash my hair for me. It was supposed to pick me up. As if getting pampered would wash any of this away.

My God, it's Valentine's Day! I never got Jeff a card or anything. The really sad thing is that it was his birthday the next day. I guess that was all the farther I got, just thinking about it. When I arrived home, I apologized to Jeff for forgetting both Valentine's Day and his birthday. I promised I would make it up to him when I felt better. This was ironic that I told him that because, I remember when it was our first anniversary and he was in Okinawa with the Marines. He called me that night and just before he hung up he told me that, "next year it would be better."

"Having you well is all the present I want," he said softly as he put his arms around me. I always felt safe in his arms.

I just cried, "I can't believe this is happening to us. Why is God punishing me, us? What awful crime had we committed? I wish someone would tell me so I could perhaps end this whole nightmare."

That evening our friend stopped by again, she said that the next day was her day off and asked if she could go with us to Rochester, we agreed. We didn't have to be there until one-thirty so we decided to not leave before nine the next morning.

My aunt didn't need to return; she found out that her memory loss was really nothing to be alarmed about. The doctors had told her that it wasn't brain cancer or anything like that; she simply was stressed out and overworked. (There is that nasty word again —STRESS. It seems to hang around like a ghost.) We were all very happy about her outcome. Tomorrow we would celebrate my diagnosis too! I felt reassured so, when I closed my eyes that night when I went to bed I didn't even need the Xanax I had been using to help me sleep.

In the morning we sent the children off to school telling them we'd see them that night when we got home. It would probably be around dinnertime because we didn't see the doctor until after lunch that day. The look on their faces was that of fear. I hugged each of them trying to reassure them that Mom would be okay.

When our friend arrived around ten we piled into our station wagon and headed north, back to Rochester. The conversation in the car was just as light as it was the day before; it was much more relaxing compared to the strain of our first day's visit. Taking the back roads my aunt showed us was sure nice; we cut off about thirty minutes from the trip instead of taking the interstate. The day was sunny again but still cold. I didn't care because I knew we were all warm and toasty inside. Both inside the car and our hearts, we knew I would beat this and then get our lives back.

Once we arrived in Rochester we decided to get something to eat. Having lived in Rochester before, our friend knew her way around the city well. We managed to find a cute little coffee shop that had great sandwiches. I must have smoked two packs of cigarettes during our lunch. Nervous habit smoking was for me! I only smoked those cancer sticks when I was either on the telephone or something made me upset. My throat still hurt and naturally my rash hadn't gone away. In fact, if I wasn't mistaken I think at least two more bumps had sprouted up overnight.

We arrived on the twelfth floor at about one, and I checked in at the desk. On the way up in the car we talked about how the people in the waiting room treated their cancers so nonchalantly. Taking our seats seeing if what we had experienced the day before might happen again. And it sure did, this tall very thin man, I guessed him to be around fifty-five began talking. "I had it in the lung, the colon and some on the liver. I was supposed to die twelve years ago and I'm still here."

"Yeah, me too, but they used some new medicine on me and I'm still in remission," another lady piped in.

It sure amazed me that they took such a positive approach to their illnesses. I decided that day this was how I wanted to face my cancer; head-on and with a positive attitude. I wasn't going to let lymphoma get me down. "Mrs. Jeanine Marsters, please." Wow, this time it didn't take long at all to get taken back to see the doctor. Jeff and I followed the nurse to the exam room waiting for the doctor to come in.

It wasn't very long before the same doctor I had the day before popped his head in. He went to the desk and dialed a number. "Yes she is here now, do you want to come up? No I haven't told her anything I thought I'd wait to tell them till you get here." He then turned to us saying, "We have to wait a few minutes so we can have the hematologist here. I told you I would consult one. I just spoke to him he'll be right up."

I was a little taken aback by this; I thought to myself, he was being somewhat mysterious. If it was what he had suspected, then why not just tell us and be done with it. Was it perhaps something else, oh no it was something else…At about the time I started to panic the door swung open to a short thin man. He was also middle-aged, graying only at the temples. He had big brown eyes and his accent wasn't exactly one I was familiar with. He seemed to study me a bit over his half rimmed glasses as if I were a laboratory rat caught in a most unpleasant trap.

He introduced himself as one of the hematologists there at the clinic, explaining how he reviewed my bone marrow test results with my doctor. This guy was a bundle of energy, I thought. I sat holding my breath. My knees I knew were going to be a sure giveaway to the level of anxiety I was feeling because they were knocking pretty bad. I needed to use my hands to steady them. I sighed and sighed again, from the corner of my eye I could see Jeff sitting straight as an arrow staring ahead.

He continued, "After careful examination of the aspirate and the biopsy, I have made the diagnosis of AML, which is acute myelogenous leukemia." It was as though I had just been sucker punched, the wind was taken out of me. I couldn't breathe without needing to gasp for air.

What? Did he just tell me I had leukemia? This couldn't be true. I am supposed to have lymphoma and I am supposed to be able to be cured. No one survives leukemia. They die! I wanted to live! I wanted to see the children grow up and get married. I wanted to see my grandchildren. Oh no, this can't be, what happens now? I suddenly felt ill. I wanted to throw up. I wanted to run away!

In the 1960s there was only a four percent chance of survival for patients with leukemia. The 70s weren't much better; in fact, during that time Jeff had worked with leukemia patients and none of them survived. The only treatment then was to put them in a sterile environment just to keep them alive as long as possible.

I finally gathered enough strength to turn to Jeff, not holding back any of the rage I was feeling inside and curtly said, "So Happy Birthday!"

With that Jeff began to tremble and sob almost uncontrollably. The tears ran down his cheeks, his face turned bright red. His worst fears seemed to be coming true. He finally let loose of all the feelings he had held back for the past week. Suddenly, I regretted what I had said. I knew I couldn't take it back though. I had hurt him deeply and I didn't know how to fix it. I didn't know if I could fix it. I reached over to him and touched his hand, and then the tears ran down my cheeks too.

"It's your birthday? I'm sorry, Mr. Marsters, but we will have to keep your wife here to begin treatment. I will admit her this afternoon. She will have a central venous catheter placed tomorrow morning in surgery so we can give her the chemotherapy she needs. We must get treatment started at once," said the hematologist.

This new doctor of mine was certainly matter-of-fact about everything. I wondered if he had any feelings. He just gave me the worst news of my life and he acted like he told me I had a hangnail. In two sentences he mentioned several things that sent chills down my spine. It was that I was going into the hospital, another was surgery and yet another was my needing chemotherapy. I didn't know then but this doctor and I were destined to have the best doctor/patient relationship I had ever known. We became friends over time. He was fantastic, but all I knew at that moment was he meant business.

My doctor at home had reassured us that it wasn't going to be leukemia, "nothing like that at all," is what he said. Boy, do I have a big surprise for you, Doc!

"I will have you check in at Rochester Methodist and I will see you over there this afternoon or evening." He stood and shook our hands, and then just as swiftly as he came in the door he left.

For a few moments we sat there trying hard to process this whole thing. The silence was broken when the other doctor spoke. "I'm sorry, Mr. and Mrs. Masters. He's a good hematologist, in fact one of the best. He has been here at the clinic for many years. I'm sure he will take good care of you." He shook our hands and with his head hanging low he left.

Jeff and I slowly rose from the couch we had been sitting on. We were both numb as we walked down the hall to the waiting room, our faces red and tear stained from the news. When we got to where our friend was sitting she looked up from her book, and then stood up waiting for us to tell her. Jeff couldn't speak so I put my arms around her and whispered, "It's leukemia. I have leukemia. I have to go to the hospital to get admitted. I need to have chemotherapy." She started to cry and embraced us both. We all just stood there hugging and crying for several minutes. This wasn't how it was supposed to turn out. It was supposed to only be lymphoma; you know the stuff I could be cured from. I felt one more time like I had taken a punch in my solar plexus.

Chapter Seven

FINALLY, WE FOUND THE STRENGTH TO walk to the elevator and push the down button. The length of time waiting for the elevators at Mayo Clinic is long; it felt like we stood there forever. Finally one arrived; there was just enough room for the three of us to climb on.

I was still trying to process the fact that this was real. I believe Jeff was thinking how was he going to go home alone to tell everyone I didn't have lymphoma, I had leukemia. I wondered to myself if he would tell them I could possibly die or if they would already know it in their hearts. I don't know how you tell an eight-year-old that his mother would not be there at night to tuck him into bed. Or tell an eleven-year-old that perhaps she would not see her mother again. I wasn't accepting this myself, how could they? I would undergo a terrible ordeal but to be honest with you, I believe Jeff had the tougher job that night. I didn't envy him at all. The only thing I did envy was that he could go home.

We went to the subway level of the Mayo Building and followed the signs that led us to the admissions department of

Rochester Methodist Hospital. If I knew that it was going to be eight weeks before I would smell the outdoors again, feel a gentle breeze on my face or even hear the city traffic I would have certainly walked outside instead of using the underground subway system, even in the cold of February.

I didn't have any idea as to how long this would all take. I did know I was going to make it through all of this. How did I know? There was something inside me that just didn't let me believe any differently. Yes I was scared, at times I still am today. I just knew then that it was not going to get me. I was going to put up one hell of a fight!

In the admitting department we found at least one hundred chairs in the waiting room. In our admitting office in our hospital there were only two chairs in the office and maybe a half of a dozen seats in the main lobby. (Naturally this has changed since then, now we have about twenty-five chairs and a few more admitting clerks.)

After an hour wait, they finally came to take Jeff and I to a small cubicle where a lady was sitting behind a computer. She asked to see any insurance cards we might have with us. I didn't have mine yet as the insurance hadn't finished being processed from my hospital, but Jeff handed her his Blue Cross card.

She made several phone calls and finally gave me an armband along with a map that directed us to the hospital lobby. Back we went through the subway system to the hospital lobby. We waited to be taken to the eighth floor, where the different Hematology units were located. An escort led us.

Yes, I said an escort, what a cool idea. They actually pay someone to run people all around the hospital to x-ray, the lab or any other part of the Mayo system that may be necessary. That way the nurses aren't being tied up doing those jobs. At home, if your patient needed to go to x-ray or to the lab usually someone from those areas had to come and get them. And if they were busy in the other departments they asked the nurse caring for the patient to do the running. If you have up to seven patients to care for you don't really have the time to run anyone around. With the amount of volume Mayo handles it sure beats tying up the staff and all the separate units to escort their patients. Suffice it to say that the Mayo Clinic has their own escort service now that ought to raise a few eyebrows when the word gets out.

When the escort arrived we headed for the BMT (Bone Marrow Transplant) unit.

I was taken to a semiprivate room. I had requested a private room, but one wouldn't be available until someone was discharged, perhaps the next day. I felt like I was being sent to prison and CANCER was the warden. If I took my chemotherapy like a good girl I might get a suspended sentence or be paroled early.

Bone Marrow Transplant, what was that? I thought to myself. Neither Jeff nor I were familiar with that procedure. Upon further investigation, we discovered you first need to have donor marrow. And just where does the donor marrow come from? It comes from a relative who is compatible, usually a sibling. In other facilities, non-related donors were being tried. *I must have learned some of this in school,* I thought. It must have been in the cancer section I tried to ignore.

I was assigned the first bed as you entered the room. The rooms were smaller than I was used to and there was no carpeting on the floor. I was used to the hospital I worked in, where every room was carpeted, that is until recently when they switched back to linoleum. A nurse handed me the usual hospital garb (hospital gown and pair of shorts) showing me a place to change.

Jeff and his cohort told me they were going to get me some essentials they thought I might need. I didn't exactly come prepared to stay. I never thought once that I would be admitted; it never even crossed my mind. Because in my mind I wasn't sick!

Here I am, I thought. I was now going to experience life from the other side of a hospital bed. This could be interesting. On my admission card and on my armband it had the initials RN after my name for all to see and for hematology residents to fear. I definitely had my own ideas about how things should and would be run. The nice thing about being in the medical field and being a patient is that I knew my patient's rights. And, I wasn't afraid to let them know I knew them either.

My nurse was very cordial and informative. She gave me all the instructions I needed in one fell swoop, but I didn't grasp it all. I felt overwhelmed by the whole ordeal. I thought back to whenever we received admissions on the floor I worked; it was somewhat the same thing. We needed to get the tasks done, such as starting the IV (intravenous line), taking a blood pressure, temperature and generally assessing each new patient. Not ever once realizing that this person lying in the bed had a lot on his or her mind and were probably not hearing a word that was being said. Just as I was at this time, she could've been speaking a foreign language for all I cared. I never heard a thing!

Sometimes patients need a moment to vent their feelings by crying, yelling or even laughing. The first lesson I learned is you can't ask a patient to possibly take all the information in that you are going to give them at first sight. Repeating instructions over several times to your patient is well advised. My nurse told me the rules regarding the BMT unit, visiting hours and meal times. She even brought in a plastic dummy chest with the central venous catheter line like the one I was going to receive the next morning.

A Hickman catheter as she called it, named after Doctor Hickman of course. I would have this piece of silicone tubing sprouting out from my chest, like a flower in spring. It would be inserted into a vein under my collarbone that leads to my heart. This is where they would run the chemotherapy through, which in turn could save my life. I did not remember one thing she said. I was too dazed.

We as nurses, along with other health care professionals, need to spend time listening to the fears and stories our patients bring with them. Maybe they are single parents or they are married and their spouse is gone someplace on business. Things like spouses, children, pets and finances are what they are really concerned about at the time of admission.

Forget the paperwork for a moment! I know for a fact, when an admission arrives on a unit and the nurses are short-handed or it's at the end of the shift, all you want to do is get the job done. Not ever concerning themselves about the patient or their feelings. It isn't intentional so don't get me wrong. We all want to be the type of nurse that is depicted in the movies. But, they have us bogged down under a ton of paperwork. It takes the completion of nine pages to get a patient admitted to a unit, which is before computerized charting came upon the scene.

It's unfortunate but sometimes nursing is more task oriented than we'd like it to be. As a student nurse I would take maybe two patients maximum in any clinical setting. We know this is idealistic, not very realistic. Most of the time you will have anywhere from six to eight patients on a team. A team at my hospital is also called a "dyad"; this is where two people, whether it is two RNs, an RN and LPN, an RN/LPN with a nursing assistant. These two people are responsible for the care of those patients in their team no matter how many of them there are, albeit two or twenty-two.

By this time my head was spinning. She had given me too much information. I think mentally, I was still back in the doctor's office in Mason City getting the news. I knew I would need many days to sort through all of this, but I didn't have the time. I would be starting chemotherapy as soon as everything was in place.

When Jeff and his shadow arrived back to my room; I was already starting to panic. I told them both I needed to get out of there. I pleaded and cried to no avail! I was beginning to feel claustrophobic, I was starting to hyperventilate and my palms were clammy. They had bought me a new pair of pajamas; they also had some stationary and stamps. "Write letters, you don't actually think I will be staying here long enough to write anyone letters, do you? My God, I don't want pen pals, I want to go home." There was also some deodorant, a toothbrush, shampoo and all the other essentials you might need to go on a vacation or stay in the hospital, but definitely not a vacation in the hospital.

Jeff said he would be back that weekend with anything else I thought I needed. I was to make a list and call him. What! This weekend, what could he be talking about; he surely wasn't leaving me here, was he? I mean our friend could take a bus home for all I cared, but Jeff needed to stay.

"You can't leave me here. I can't go through this alone," I sobbed.

"Bun (a private nickname we gave each other when we first were married and it has stuck ever since), I have to take care of the kids. I have to go and tell them what has happened," he said, trying to fight back his tears, with very little success.

"Jeff, please don't leave me here, I am scared," I cried. Just then the doctor came into the room. She was the Chief Resident on the hematology service. She had in tow one of her fledglings. One who would be assigned to my case. As time went on I discovered that the residents rotated through the hematology area every two weeks. Mayo Clinic is a teaching facility so it is overrun with residents. I thought to myself, *All residents beware; I have them for breakfast at home.*

They asked Jeff to step out while they examined me, it would only take a few moments, they said. We joked through the entire exam. Finally, they must've noticed my pensive state coming back because one of them looked at me and said, "It isn't anything that you did, believe me it wasn't the cigarettes you smoked in the girls bathroom while you were in high school that brought you here, it just happened. Don't blame yourself, you couldn't have prevented this." Was that a relief? How did they know I had been doing just that, blaming myself for this dreaded disease? *If I hadn't smoked perhaps I would not be here now*, I thought. I finally took a look at these doctors and knew I was among friends. I still wanted to go home.

The Chief Resident was quite plain, but a beautiful person to me nonetheless. She had long medium brown hair, which she kept pulled back with a large barrette. She wore a herringbone suit, which clung, smartly to her slight figure. She couldn't have been more than five feet tall, in heels. She wore no makeup and spoke with a slight lisp. A real giant in my eyes, through the next few weeks she would also become my confidante. Someone I could share all my fears and dreams with.

71

"I know you will be just fine," she said with a smile and put her arm around me. "I will let your husband spend some time with you and I will come back later." With that she exited my room taking her young resident with her.

I could see them standing outside my room talking to Jeff. I was a little annoyed by that. *They better not be holding anything back from me*, I thought to myself. That was one thing I insisted on, tell me everything, I may need time to process it but don't hold anything back. Finally, Jeff shook their hands, smiled and came back into my room.

I asked, a little sarcastically, "What were you talking about?" He had such a confused look on his face. I apologized for acting like a bitch, but I was afraid that I would not be included on things that concerned me. My control over things was being taken away but I wanted to be in charge of my own destiny.

After all, I was a nurse and I knew that sometimes doctors would try to spare their patient by not always being totally honest with them. They would always tell the family everything. Or the family would tell the doctors to not tell everything to the patient. I wanted no part of that kind of thinking, I wanted the whole truth and nothing but the truth. No matter how bad it was. So help me God! After a few more moments of silence Jeff finally said the doctors called me "Spunky."

Spunky, well that must be a nicer term for bitch I guess. But that didn't matter; I would be as spunky or bitchy as I needed to be, because you see I will survive! No leukemia would get me or get me down either.

I really didn't want to be alone though. Loneliness was something I dealt with too much as a young child. Lonely was how I felt when I lost my brother one summer day at the age of nine. Lonely was how I felt while I was in the Navy transferring from one duty station to another. Lonely was how I felt when Jeff was shipped overseas to Okinawa for six months leaving Jennifer and I alone. Now here I again had to face lonely one more time.

The nights were what I discovered to be my hardest. I never realized how long the darkness of night lasted. I didn't like the isolation from my husband, my children and from all those I loved. Now they were going to put me up here away from everyone to fight this disease alone. I didn't realize I was not alone; I had God and the angels watching over and comforting me.

I finally got over my stubbornness realizing that Jeff had to leave to be with our children. He had to go home, to tell them Mom was sicker than anyone believed. Before he departed they gave me the best pick me up he could have found. A calendar on which I could mark off the days of my stay and a calendar of hunks! These were some of the most beautiful male bodies I had ever seen. They were clad in these little bikinis, you know *SPEEDO*'s. Oh yeah, that was definitely my kind of calendar. He had also gotten me a black felt tip pen to mark off the days until I could return home.

This was only to be a small detour, a bend in the road so to speak. It was hard to see him go. I couldn't stop crying for a long while after he left. I did wait to start though until he was out of sight, then I let the floodgates open. The staff was sensitive enough to realize I simply needed to be alone for a while...I needed time to reflect on all the things I had learned these past few days. I needed to get in touch with my spiritual side...

Chapter Eight

THE ROOMMATE I HAD WAS AN elderly confused lady. This was my lucky day, I thought to myself. She lay in her bed picking at something she thought she saw in the air. All I could do was shake my head; I got up to draw the curtain that separated us, keeping her on her half of the room and me on my side. I was not in the mood for socializing anyway. I definitely needed a private room.

I found the remote for the TV on the bed rail and began channel-surfing aimlessly. There were many more channels to choose from than what we could receive in our hospital, for that I was thankful. I finally found *The Bill Cosby Show* and settled down to watch thirty minutes of life with the Huxtables. I wonder how Cliff would have handled leukemia, I thought to myself. Or do they even get leukemia on TV? Could it be funny?

I found myself laughing uncontrollably during this episode. It was the one where Theo decides he is going to live in the real world. So, his mom and dad used monopoly money to show him what it would really be like. It was a great episode and for those thirty minutes I actually forgot my own problems.

It was then that I decided I only wanted to watch funny shows and funny movies. If it could work for Norman Cousins to ease his pain I would use it for myself to survive cancer, what did I have to lose? So humor therapy became part of my own medical regimen: chemotherapy, vomiting, hair loss, nausea, diarrhea and a lot of laughter, what a prescription! When you get done with the formula you have a LIFE. I'll let you in on a little secret; it has worked this far so I will continue to laugh in the face of adversity, or as I called it when I was young, atrocity. You don't have to be faced with cancer or any other life-threatening disease to look at life with a little more sense of humor.

The doctor returned later that night to explain to me about the Hickman I would be getting in the morning. She sat there on the edge of my bed speaking softly telling me that there was nothing to worry about because they would take good care of me. Her voice was relaxing and her sincerity was almost overwhelming. She told me she would leave an order for a sleeping pill for me that night if I thought I needed it. I only nodded; just what I want to start doing was using sleeping pills. Remember I was from the generation that Jacqueline Susan's novel *Valley of the Dolls* was about back in the 1960s, so I felt well informed about the use of "dolls." I realized I could do this without medication, I thought to myself. I can be tough and strong. As the night went on I realized I should have taken the drugs.

As I lay in the darkness trying desperately to sleep but couldn't; I saw the hours tick by on my watch comparing it to the clock on the wall. I would pretend to be sleeping, as the night nurses would scurry in and out of the room, trying to not engage in any senseless conversation. I wanted to be left alone to think, to reflect on the day's events. They were kept busy most of the night anyway with my roommate, stopping by my bed only long enough to remove my water pitcher shortly after midnight. You see going to surgery in the morning required me to be NPO, which means "nothing by mouth." Being a surgical nurse I was quite familiar with the routine.

Just then my roommate got up and went to the bathroom. I

guess I didn't think of any reason why she shouldn't have been up alone until I heard a thud come from behind the closed door. I called for the nurse. She entered our room almost immediately. I told her I thought my roommate might have fallen in the bathroom. Her eyes grew wide with fright and ran to the bathroom trying to open the door, but couldn't because the patient was apparently leaning against it after her fall. She went out to get more help.

When she and another nurse returned to the room they tried the door again. They were shouting to the woman lying in the bathroom. Asking her whether or not she was OK. The bathrooms were very small in these rooms. The stool and a sink left not enough room to maneuver in there if someone fell. They finally worked on the door making it swing out instead of in and were able to rescue the lady on the floor. Just as I thought, she now seemed to be even more confused. I could hear them scolding her like a child for getting out of her bed without calling for help behind the drawn curtain.

One of them stopped momentarily at the foot of my bed before exiting. She was a tall girl with short dark brown hair. "Thanks for calling when you did. I think she will be okay now," she said.

"I'm sorry I didn't call before she fell but I didn't know she couldn't be up," I said apologetically.

"You couldn't have known. Is there anything you need?" she said with a smile.

"Yes. I could really use that sleeping pill the doctor ordered for me. I haven't slept much," I said, turning and looking toward the curtain that separated me from the little lady who was picking things out of the air.

"I'm sorry but it's three in the morning and it's too late to give a sleeping pill to you now." With that she left the room and joined the other nurse who had been in to help her. They were giggling and gesturing, so I knew they were discussing the incident that had just occurred. They finally walked away from the window so I couldn't see them anymore.

A tear slid down my cheek, three in the morning, what was I to do until the sun came up? *Oh, God, please help me*, I prayed. *I haven't been the greatest one for prayer but I am doing it now, help me to get through this.* Isn't it interesting we always call on God when the going gets tough; we forget to thank Him when life is great?

I hated this place; I hated my body for doing this to me. *Why? What did I do, God, that you did this to me? I thought that if I did everything right and never hurt anyone then nothing bad would happen.* Besides hadn't I already suffered enough in my life? Let someone else suffer for a while. I had to wait until the morning when I would go to surgery to begin my fight.

Chapter Nine

"MRS. MARSTERS," SOMEONE SAID, TOUCHING MY leg gently. I looked up to see a young man dressed in surgical garb. I found out later he was an orderly. I must have fallen asleep. The last time I looked at the clock it was four-thirty, and now it was seven. I thought for a moment and smiled, *Thanks, God, for taking away the night*. No more of this, I was going to take a sleeping pill every night I was in this place. I needed to sleep this all away if I could. I believe that sleeping in the hospital is near to impossible. As I remembered back, not many patients slept through the night without some kind of disruption.

"Mrs. Marsters?" the young man repeated.

"Yes, I am Mrs. Marsters," I said as I stretched my arms upwards for a minute. Stretching just like a cat waking from a nap.

"I'm here to take you to surgery," he continued. There he stood with my chart in hand and a surgical cart behind. My chart, boy I can remember many times when patients wanted to read their charts and what a big deal it was. They would need clearance from their doctors before they could read it. I even believe they checked with the Pope! Now being a patient myself, I too was curious. I wanted to know what they had written in there. Did they write that I slept peacefully through the night? Wouldn't that be a laugh, seeing as I was awake for most of it, and lucky for them I was. If I hadn't been up, how long would my roommate have lain on the bathroom floor before someone found her?

I got up and slowly walked over to the surgical cart and climbed aboard. Many times I had put patients on these hard, narrow carts sending them merrily off to the operating room. If this whole ordeal was supposed to be some kind of a lesson about being a better nurse, then I had better take notes. If this was to be a lesson in humility, then consider me humbled. I promised myself to not forget any of these experiences. This was when I started journaling, writing down everything daily about how I felt, what treatment I was having, and even my hopes and dreams... these were my most inner thoughts.

I never knew what a nauseating experience it was to be wheeled down hospital corridors on a cart. The lights on the ceilings passing overhead made me feel like I was spinning. I closed my eyes for most of the ride trying to avoid throwing up on the nice clean sheets I was on.

Finally reaching our destination, the holding area. This is where everyone stops just before entering surgery. This is where they check your records to make sure they are intact and to confirm that you are actually Mr. Smith or Mrs. Jones. Or Mrs. Marsters in my case. They will perform a hernia and not a mastectomy or a Hickman placement and not a knee replacement. The final checkpoint so to speak before the adventure begins.

I was greeted by a friendly smile from a holding area nurse. She was wearing green scrubs and had the neatest surgical cap on her head. "Where did you get that cap?" I asked her, pointing to her head.

"One of the nurses here makes them." She smiled with a puzzled look on her face. The hat was one of many colors, neon green and had frogs on it. The surgeons in our hospital now wear multicolored scrub caps; they were just a little behind. For now it was the neatest one I had ever seen. She told me that a nurse who worked in the holding area made them for the staff.

"Seeing as I will be bald soon, after I start my chemotherapy, I will be in the market for some unusual head wraps," I said jokingly.

With that she laughed. "Let me get her name for you and maybe she will make you some, they are only two dollars. At least that is what she charges us, maybe they will be more for you, and heck you can always try asking her." With that she turned and left my side, after patting me on the head. I never did see her after that, and I never did buy any of the scrub hats, I got into scarves instead.

I have always recommended the book *Beauty and Cancer* written by Peggy Mellody, RN and Diane Doan-Noyes to my patients (that is until now, I have learned it is out of print). Maybe you can still find it in a library. In the book is a section about hair alternatives. The entire book has valuable information for women undergoing cancer therapy. Beauty and cancer are two words we don't see used together yet alone in the same sentence.

The cancer units at Rochester Methodist hospital have a copy of this on each of the floors. At times they gave their patients copies too. And if all else failed they had it in the hospital library. This will help transform you to the new you in several different ways. It has makeup tips, how to make scarves, how to dress, how to select wigs and a lot more. It was a start before I found *Look Good Feel Good.*

Now there is a program *Look Good Feel Good,* sponsored by the ACS (American Cancer Society) where they provide cosmetologists, wig stylists, makeup along with skin care tips. You can find out anything else that could help to make you *Look Good Feel Good.* This was really a psychological boost, we all need when facing the changes in our bodies, especially women.

Before leaving the hospital I was approached by a woman that was involved in the starting up of the *Look Good Feel Good* in Rochester. She wanted to know if I would preview the information about the program. She wanted to know whether or not it would be a useful program to start. Wow! What an honor it was to be asked. I gave her the old thumbs up!

You should see the group now. It has blossomed into this marvelous opportunity for women to learn how to still look good without eyelashes. That one always puzzled me. They provide each person a box full of beauty supplies and then they have local cosmetologists to help you use it all. They even sell wigs, scarves and head wraps. To this day this woman talks about a cancer patient who helped her get it all started. What a testimony to my fight, I thought.

Someone approached me from the anesthesia department next. He explained that this procedure was going to be done under a local anesthetic. He promised to make me comfortable during the procedure. A surgical resident who again explained the entire surgery to me followed him. I just wanted to get the damn thing done! Continuously going over the procedure only made me more anxious.

The surgical resident was funny even though I was nervous, he made me start to feel a little more relaxed. As I lay there waiting for my turn I looked down the row of surgical carts to see twenty-five or so people lying there waiting to go into surgery. Amazing!

As a graduate nurse when I visited our holding area to learn how to start IVs I noticed that there were only five carts for patients and only two were filled. I started listening to one lady slurring her speech a bit after they had given her some medicine to relax her before heading in for cataract surgery. Even though I never considered being a recovery or surgical nurse it was fun to listen to the hustle and bustle. I always have preferred my patients awake.

When they finally came to take me into surgery, they assured me it wasn't going to take too long. Once the procedure was over I would go to the recovery room for about thirty minutes and then back to my room.

"So you're a nurse," the guy wheeling my cart said. "What's your flavor? What should we give you? It will be a local, but we will relax you. We can give you enough medication so you do actually go to sleep if you want." He laughed at that.

"Let's put it this way," I told him. "Put me far enough under that I won't remember anything or be aware you're even here, but not so far that I would need to be intubated." With that everyone in the surgical suite laughed.

That was the last thing I remember until I awoke in the recovery room. I was feeling a little stiff and my shoulder did hurt a bit. In fact the longer I lay there the more the whole left side of my chest hurt. I was afraid to look down to see what they had done to me.

"Everything is finished, Mrs. Marsters. I am just waiting for the orderly to return you to your room," this voice said coming from behind me. I looked over the end of my cart backwards to see a rather plumpish white-haired lady sitting in a chair writing on a chart. Tipping my head so far back made me a little queasy, so I stopped trying to see the person talking to me. How rude, I thought, you could have at least gotten yourself up to talk to me, not shout at me from across the room.

I gazed down the row again to see many carts, there must have been fifteen people lying on them. Some were being monitored, some were throwing up and some had to be held down because they were out of control from the effects of having anesthesia. *Ah! The life of the recovery room*, I thought to myself, this wasn't a place I wanted to ever work. It takes a quick nurse to monitor those changes that occur in the recovery room, besides not every patient does well. It is a real test of one's nursing skills. Somehow I derived more pleasure being able to communicate with my patients.

The same young man who had brought me down to this icebox was suddenly there to take me back. I would be happy to get back to my room because I was freezing. I believe that the temperature in surgical area ranges ever so slightly between Alaska and the North Pole. Cold is a mild term to use. An icebox would be a more fitting term. We started back down the halls swiftly. On the way back I automatically closed my eyes the entire way.

The ride back seemed to be a lot faster, why is that? When we arrived on the unit again, I had by some miracle been moved to a private room. I never did see my confused roommate again nor did I ask what became of her. I had too many things occupying both my mind and time in the days and weeks ahead to worry about such things.

The cart came to a stop outside the door to my new home. I got off thanking the young man for the ride and walked into my room. I couldn't believe my eyes, a room all to myself, I could be alone and not worry about my roommate's family members stopping at the foot of my bed each time they entered to visit. I was in no mood to make idle chitchat with total strangers.

I was in quite a mood though. First I was in pain, hard to be upbeat when you hurt like hell. The next thing I felt was violation. I felt that the Hickman was in a way an insult to my body being imposed on me because of this damn disease. Some other feelings I had were of being stunned, sorrow, fear, confusion…the list could go on. It is easier to simply say I had an attitude!

Chapter Ten

THE VIEW FROM MY WINDOW WAS not much to behold, with only bricks to look at, but it was my view. I could watch the comings and goings of the Rochester Canadian geese that lived at Silver Lake, which was not too far from the hospital. They would leave in their V-formations every morning and arrive back home in the late afternoon. Such freedom they had, I thought. I formed a close attachment to them from a distance, from my window. I longed for the days when I too could fly, to be free from this disease, to be whole again. For now I was sprouting this foreign object from my left breast, my Hickman, my central venous catheter. This is the thing that would bring me both treatment and life over the next several months.

Just as I stood at the window watching the geese my nurse entered the room interrupting my thoughts. "What do you see out there?" she asked.

"Nothing," I replied. "Just watching the world go by," I said, smiling to myself.

"Are you feeling okay? Do you need anything? I need you to get into bed, so I can check your Hickman site." With that she pointed to my bed as she drew back the covers.

I obliged by walking over and climbing in. I glanced back out the window at the geese one more time as the sun set. My shoulder was tender and stiff, but I managed to tolerate it. I must remember to thank those nice boys in surgery, I thought, they did their job well. I didn't recall any of the goings-on in the operating room. *Thank you, God,* I thought, looking upward.

She leaned over and pulled my gown down to expose my new tubes. It didn't look as bad as I thought it might, there was a long white silicone tube that split in two a third of the way down. At the end were two small caps attached. Just before the caps were two clamps that were there to stop the flow of fluid when not in use. It was truly ugly and I hated it. The tubes themselves served two purposes; I was able to receive fluids and also be saved from the numerous blood draws I needed. Perhaps I would get used to it, but for now I just wanted it covered up so I didn't have to look at it.

After the nurse inspected the new site she left. I was again alone with my thoughts and I could feel an all too familiar tear give way and begin to roll down my cheek. I turned to face the window quickly so no one walking past my room would see. To watch the geese fly by, to dream...to sleep. I remember reading that in my psychology book while I was in school. Depression leads to many more hours of sleep. One sleeps to escape the reality of what is happening around you or to you.

I was awakened by the voice of a young woman. She told me she was the diet assistant, she was very tall, thin, with dark brown curly shoulder length hair. She wore glasses and had a bright smile. "Here's your evening meal, Jeanine," she said. "I hope everything is to your liking. If there is anything different I can get you, please let me know." With that she turned and exited.

Diet assistants do two things, one was to free the nursing staff of the duties while they dealt with critical patients and two there aren't enough dietitians to go around to help everyone with their meals. These gals took the pressure off of everyone. Their uniforms were black pants or skirts, white shirts and burgundy vests. It's a uniform that distinguished them from the ward secretaries or escorts who had navy blue vests, white shirts and navy blue pants.

The phone rang; the beds have many things attached to the side rails; the TV controls, the bed controls and the telephone. I grew to like the idea as I picked up the receiver. "Hi!" the voice said; it was Jeff calling me before he went home from work.

"Hello," I replied.

"I was glad to hear you have a private room," he continued.

"How did you know I was moved to a private room?"

"I called earlier, you were still down in surgery and they told me then you would be moved." He sounded so depressed. I wanted desperately to see his face and to look into his eyes. I wanted him to hold me. I tried to fight back the tears, but was unable to. I seemed to cry more than I ever had before, partly out of fear and being separated from the people I loved. Either way, I had cried a river of tears.

"Gig, are you okay?" he asked, his voice sounding concerned. (Gigi was a nickname I gave myself when I was a little girl and couldn't say Jeanine.)

"Yeah, I guess it's just that this thing is so ugly that they put in me, it sticks out and I hate it," I blurted out. "Make this all go away!"

"If it will make you better, that's all that counts, isn't it?" he asked. I couldn't argue with that logic. I stopped crying, I have learned after many years of marriage, nothing irritated Jeff more than for me to cry. It made him feel helpless and feeling helpless made him angry.

"I told the kids," he continued.

"What did they say?" I asked. My poor babies, I thought, trying once again to fight back the tears.

"What do you think they said? Jennifer started to cry and Justin just ran crying to his room. They are afraid; they don't want you to die. I also called their teachers and talked to them too. I asked them to watch for any behaviors they might see. I thought they could help."

"Don't you think that was a little too much?" I asked.

"No I don't, I have to deal with this at home and I think that this will help them in the long run. Those teachers can watch to see if there is anything we need to catch early. This is hard for them and they need to know that their teachers care. I also talked to the kids' sitter. They couldn't believe it, especially after their niece was diagnosed with leukemia four months earlier." She stood a chance of a cure, her doctors said, if she stayed in remission long enough for the cure to work. She was too weak, the chemotherapy was hard on her and her disease was strong. She passed away in the fall of 1990, at the age of fourteen; she fought her battle with cancer bravely.

"Jeanine, are you still there?" he asked with concern.

I had drifted away momentarily deep in thought. "Yeah, I'm here," I replied. "It's so strange that now I have leukemia too, don't you think? Just tell them all of them to take good care of my babies," I said with tears welling up in my eyes.

"Listen, I have to go, it's time to go home and pick up the kids." Jeff again brought me back to the present. I couldn't believe it was time to hang up; I wanted to stay on the line forever. I didn't want to go back to the loneliness.

"Do you have to go?" I asked. "Can't we just talk a little longer?"

"No, I have to go. I'll call you in the morning, okay? If you need me just call me! But, if you can wait until I get to work then do, I'll try to call from work a couple of times each day." With that we said our good-byes and hung up.

Sometimes he could be too mater-of-fact for my liking. When I thought about it later I understood why, he was trying to keep it all together. I needed to keep in mind he had to deal with much more than my loneliness or my Hickman catheter. He simply needed to keep a clear head.

I sat there for a long while just holding on to the receiver. It was the buzzing of the phone that brought me back down to earth. I had left it off the hook. My mind kept wandering, it would go back to a time when I was well and life was better. I decided then I wasn't going to get beaten by cancer, I was going to make it and with the help of God I would take my life back! My babies needed me and so did Jeff!

The rest of the evening I just paced around my room looking out of the window. Time seemed to drag on. The only interruption was that of the night nurse, as she would move in and out to check on me. The shifts were split into two twelve-hour shifts instead of the traditional three eight-hour shifts that I was familiar with, the new shift began at seven. They were all very nice and their little interruptions were oftentimes welcomed.

I learned a long time ago that there are no strangers in the world, only friends we hadn't met yet. This was true of the staff that took care of me. We became great friends during the times I was in their care. I learned a lot about caring for my patients from them. These angels of mercy never batted an eye when we would often talk for hours. They never left if I needed them, always listening to my fears as well as my dreams. These nurses were the Florence Nightingales of the 1990s and they were my heroes.

Chapter Eleven

THE NEXT MORNING WAS FILLED WITH more of the same kind of waiting. I was still trying to get used to my surroundings. In the late morning I had visitors from home, a couple of nurses I worked with. It was good to see them, but there seemed to be a cloud hanging over our visit. Everyone was nice, perhaps a little too nice, we were all so afraid what was going to happen to me next. No one wanted to talk about what was going on for fear if they talked about it, reality would sink in and it would become true. We did laugh a lot though; as we chatted about the floor we worked on, our families and friends.

Finally, the seriousness of this situation seemed to bring us back to earth when I showed them my Hickman. We talked about the days to come. When they came to take me down to have some tests done the girls decided to head for home. We all cried as we said good-bye. Then I left by wheelchair to see another doctor, believe it or not, to have another pap smear. They certainly run you through all kinds of tests, making sure you are clear of everything before they start the treatment process.

Every woman knows the thrill of a pap smear, so you all know how much I wanted to have that done, especially since I had just had one done in December. I don't like them every year so two in three months was overkill as far as I was concerned.

When I was returned to my room it was lunchtime. I must say I was even beginning to like the food here. *I must be sick*, I thought. At least it was better than what was served at the hospital back home. I often wondered where they got their recipes. It is hard to believe there was that many ways to prepare chicken.

During our last conversation, I asked Jeff to get in touch with our pastor. I wanted to see him. He had been out of town during this time and I wanted to talk to him as soon as he returned. That afternoon I was granted my wish with a visit from him. I can't tell you how his strength carried me through. He was a different kind of pastor from the ones I remembered as a child. He never gave the hell, fire and brimstone sermons. You know what I mean, the kind where you had the fear of God preached to you each Sunday, as they would pound their fists on the pulpit. It always scared the hell out of me.

This pastor cracked Norwegian jokes, ate Lutefisk, liked treats, smiled all the time and gave great hugs. He reminded me more of a gentle loving father. His face always beaming brightly, almost like Santa. I guess that is why I wanted to see him now. I was looking desperately for answers and I was positive he had them.

"I needed to see you. Thanks for coming. I know you are busy," I said with tears streaming down my cheeks.

"I was performing a wedding, so I was out of town," he replied.

"I have so many questions I need to ask." He sat patiently beside me in a chair as I sat Indian style on the bed. "Why did this happen to me?"

"I don't know," he answered. I was shocked; when my brother died I remember that the minister we had at the time seemed to have all the answers. This kindly gentleman didn't have any he said. "Sometimes we don't understand God's plan for us."

"That's another thing, when I found out that I had cancer the first thing I did was get mad at God. I couldn't believe after all the suffering I thought that I had done in my life; he was doing this to me now. What had I done? I always thought that I was a good person, why was I being punished now?" I questioned.

Pastor just sat there listening, he let me get it all out, to vent both my pain and my sorrow. He finally talked about Job, who had his faith tested in his life by all the terrible things that had happened to him. He also gave me some other scripture verses to cling to, and then he cried with me. He told me, "God will be there to help you through. We are never alone. Lean on Him and He will carry you through this terrible time." I found peace and strength that day. Before Pastor left, he told me of a book titled *Why Do Bad Things Happen to Good People*. He said he had a copy of it and that he would find a way to get it to me.

No one had the answers. No one truly knows the mysteries of God. He then offered me communion, I took it and we prayed. He gave me a hug before he left. He'll never know how much he meant to me that day. I had always had faith in God, but I don't think it was ever as strong as it was that day.

I was becoming a bed potato instead of the traditional couch potato for many reasons, one of them being I had no couch. The door burst open that afternoon and in shot my hematologist, all five-foot-seven of him. Boy, he commanded your attention whenever he entered a room.

"Well, Mrs. Marster," he started. He leaves off the last "s" in my last name. To this day he has never gotten my last name right, he usually uses last names, after all we had been through together he rarely calls me Jeanine. "The tests are all done and we will start chemo tonight if that is agreeable with you," he said.

What do you mean agreeable, I am being held captive here with no ransom demand in sight. Now you ask if is agreeable to me. After all the poking and prodding you've done now you are thinking of whether or not I would agree. He did kind of stir something in me though; he had just the right edge to send me into orbit. It was though we had this comedy routine going on like *Abbott and Costello*. I have yet to figure out who was *Abbott* and who was *Costello*.

"By the way do you have a project to do with you?" he asked. A project, what did he mean by that? "I have all my patients while they are in here do a project; in fact, they cannot go home until they complete their projects. Do you have a project? I have three children you perhaps could make them moccasins or something." What was he talking so fast about, he expected me to make him something. For what the sheer pleasure of it? He continued. "You have your husband bring you in a project when he comes to see you I will not let you leave until that is done."

He is a wild man, I thought, now he not only is going to send chemicals through my veins, but he wants me to make him something. "What kind of project?" I was finally able to ask.

"Oh, anything, what do you do? I had one man paint me a picture, someone else stitched me a picture. Anything will do, but you will be here for a while and you need to keep your mind busy."

"You mean a hobby?" I asked. "I do counted cross-stitch."

"Good, I'll expect you to be doing that then. When your husband comes have him bring you a project to do." With that he turned and left, I thought he was crazy; he actually expected that I would make him a picture.

When Jeff called, I told him about this crazy man who now wanted me to make a cross-stitch picture. He laughed and said he'd see what he could do. He also said he'd be up to see me in the morning. Now I felt like a kid waiting for a birthday party, I was so excited to see Jeff that I was beside myself. I couldn't wait until the weekend!

Chapter Twelve

MY MOTHER CALLED LATER THAT AFTERNOON to tell me that our hairdresser would be coming up in the morning to cut my hair. The thought of going bald with the long flowing mane of hair I had now was too much to deal with. I decided that I would get my hair cut short so it wouldn't be as much of a shock when I lost it all. I had asked my mother to get in touch with our hairdresser to see if he would come up and perhaps give me a trim. And he was nice enough to agree to it.

The rest of the evening was uneventful as I waited for my chemotherapy to start. It was ten o'clock when the Chief Resident finally came to see me. "I have a form here for you to sign. This will give your consent to be followed in a study the clinic is doing on treatments for different types of cancers. It will allow us to use random selection to make the choice as to which protocol we will use for your treatment."

A computer making the choice as to which therapy I was to receive scared me a little bit. A little like Russian roulette, don't you think? It is known that computers have made mistakes before. I found it remarkable that human thought would be cast aside and a machine would decide how to treat me. We've come a long way, baby! "Is this okay?" I asked her. "Do others do this?"

"Yes, usually everyone does this, which is how we track progress of different kinds of treatments," she replied. I have grown to trust her and knew that she wouldn't let anything happen to me, so I signed the paper. Then I looked her square in the eyes and asked her if I would be able to walk in Grandma's marathon. I then explained it was a marathon named after a restaurant in Duluth, Minnesota. She told me she didn't see why not, I told her that it was good because I never could before. With that we both laughed.

I waited a few more hours until the computer made the choice before I could receive my first dose of what I still refer to as intravenous *Janitor in the Drum*. The thought of that made me even more restless than I already was.

"Boy, you keep late hours," I told her as she entered my room later that night. She still had her wool suit on that she had worn all day. Along with high heels, boy my aching feet, I thought to myself. Could my doctor be a superhero? She was to me!

"We have received the computer results." She then told me there were two different protocols that they could choose from that have been used in the past to treat my type of leukemia. One was the "tried and true method" as she referred to it, the one that has been around for many years and they have had much success with it. The other was a newer version, and that hadn't been around for more than four or five years. What this amounted to was the way in which I would receive the chemo. Hit hard in the beginning, and then have all rounds followed shortly thereafter, or stretch it out over a longer period of time. "The computer selected the 'tried and true method' for you. So we will get started as soon as the pharmacy has it ready."

"I'm afraid. Will I die?" I finally brought myself to ask the question I had not asked since I was diagnosed. I just thought if I didn't ever say the words, then it wouldn't happen. I never turned on the light in my room when she came in so there we stood in the darkness, only the light from the nurse's station shining in on us. This way she couldn't see my face or read the fear on it. But I still could see her clearly in the shadows. I could read her expression and yet she couldn't see me.

"If I had to have leukemia this would be one of the types I would choose. Not that any of them are good mind you." I felt she was being honest with me. I had come to a point in my life that I can read people pretty well, and I knew in my heart she wasn't just giving me the usual line of bull.

"Thank you," I said and shook her hand. We stood there talking for almost two hours in the darkness. It was midnight when they finally delivered my chemotherapy and she left my room. During our visit we talked about my children, my disease, my doctor and my dreams for the future. She never gave me more information than I asked for, not filling my head with a lot of mumble jumble.

Doctors often talk a kind of gibberish when they can't find the right words to say after telling patients their prognoses. They don't seem to realize that all they need to do is listen to the patients; they will help you find the words to say. Allow them to take the opportunity to express exactly what is on their minds. Just tell us in words we can understand, "keep it simple." Too much information going in and not enough time to process it all.

The nurse broke in on our conversation when she came in the room with some medication and an IV bag. I could feel my heart race and my palms get sweaty. *My God*, I thought, *it's really going to happen, I will never be the same again after this.* I knew that much for sure! She was startled by the fact the good doctor and I were standing in the dark talking, so when she came through the door she gasped a little. "Oh, you scared me!" she said. "I thought you were asleep and now I find you guys having a party in here without me." She looked at the doctor. "I thought you had gone home hours ago, I didn't know you were in here."

"Were you looking for me? Did you need something?" she asked.

"No, I just thought you had gone home," she said. She then

95

turned her attention to me, as she continued. "I have some pre-medication to give you. It helps to stop some of the side effects of the chemotherapy. It won't take care of them totally, but it will make it somewhat more tolerable." I can't remember for sure if it was just Ativan, Benadryl or Compazine or all three of them. Who cares it did the trick. In fact, I do believe I slept through most of the administration of my first round of chemotherapy.

"Is that it in there?" I asked, pointing to the IV bag she had in her hand.

Before she left the doctor cupped my shoulder in her hand and said good night, she'd see me in the morning. "You'll do just fine," she said and left the room.

"Yes, this is the continuous drip of Ara-C, the other chemotherapy drug you'll be given is called Daunorubicin. That is an IV push drug; the Ara-C will run for three days, every twelve hours for an hour. We will continue to give you pre-medications to help you through."

"I guess we need to get this show on the road, right?" I said and hopped into bed. She hung some other IV fluid first with which she ran the premeds through. I could feel the warm flush run through my body, and felt that sleep wouldn't be too far off. The last thing I remember that night was that she was connecting the bag of chemotherapy to my Hickman. I closed my eyes shortly after that and slept peacefully until morning.

When I awoke I didn't feel much different, until I started to get up, the bones in my ankles ached when I first tried to walk. Chemotherapy side effects. I had to go to the bathroom, I remember that the nurse had told me to not be frightened if my urine turned red, that was one of the side effects of the Daunorubicin. I was glad she told me that because; I almost fainted when I stood up and found bright red urine. With that also came my first wave of nausea, and I hurried to get back to my bed. Surprisingly enough, I didn't throw up. If this was all there was to it, then it wouldn't be so bad, I thought.

Later that morning my hairdresser showed up and did the dastardly deed, he cut my long curly locks off. I was now one cropped chicken. I hated short hair; I always thought my ears were too big. It was only going to get worse; it wouldn't be long before I lost my hair altogether. I didn't know that as time went on I would resent people that had hair.

I used to make fun of a friend while I was in nursing school about her having wimpy hair, little did I know I would have wimpier thin fine hair than she ever did when this was all done. We laughed as we always did whenever he cut my hair. There was a certain sadness that came to both of us as he swept up the golden tresses from my hospital room floor. Bending down only to salvage a few strands to take with him, to use in matching a wig for me.

A wig, how funny I thought, I remember when I used to harass my mother when she wore wigs back in the 1960s. Even though at the time it was quite fashionable. Now, I would be able to wear the wig in the family. My impression of wigs was not good; to me they looked phony, perched on top of someone's head like a bird's nest or a rug as they are sometimes referred to. That is probably why I never came to wear the silly thing, I opted to adorn myself in flowery head wraps of my own design instead.

I thanked him before he left, and went into the bathroom. I stared at myself in the mirror as the tears began falling from my eyes uncontrollably. My God, what have you done to me? My hair, cut short, gone forever! My body, well that was failing me too, I thought. It was against me as it allowed this disease to overtake it. I looked down at the tube coming from my chest and really began to sob. How can I go through this? Will the horror of it all ever end?

Suddenly, I was jolted back from my thoughts as a voice came from inside my room. "Gig, where are you?" It was Jeff; he had come for his weekend visit. He was going to stay at the hotel across from the hospital. He didn't have the children with him this time; he came alone.

"I'll be right out," I shouted back at him. My face was pretty red now and I was not looking forward to a lecture from him about my crying, so I desperately tried to throw cold water on it.

I always cried at everything, including after sex. Don't get me wrong, Jeff wasn't an ogre, he just didn't like to see me upset. It upset him when I cried but this was a situation he couldn't fix. It was out of both of our hands, we had to just go through it.

"You've been crying," he said. He put his arms out and gave me a hug, that didn't help matters any as I really began to cry then. "Stop!" he said, as my body was now quacking under his embrace.

"What are we going to do?" I asked. Pulling away from him and looking into his eyes. They say that the eyes are the windows to the soul. Looking into Jeff's eyes that day I could only see the sorrow and fear of what was ahead for us, for him alone possibly. We had no guarantees or any ideas as to if this would work. I just kept telling myself that I would get through it.

"We will take one day at a time, that's all we can do." He sat down in a chair next to the bed as I sat on the bed. We talked for quite awhile as we watched TV. Lunch came and Jeff decided that he would go and get himself something to eat. He would leave my room from time to time to smoke a cigarette in the Kahler Hotel cafeteria.

You must meet my husband, or perhaps you already have and didn't know it. He is noted for his friendliness. He will walk up to total strangers and before the end of a conversation they would be laughing and joking like they were old friends. I can't tell you how many times I would ask him how long he knew someone he had been talking to and he would laugh telling me he'd just met the guy.

He is great in the neighborhood we live in because all the little old ladies think he's super. He will do anything for them, so while I was in the hospital he would make many of these journeys to the Kahler and met many interesting people. Lord love him!

It was infuriating whenever I had dinner waiting at home. He would be late because he was helping one of the neighbors. Recently, I was in a grocery store in town, Jeff let me out at the door so I wouldn't get wet in the rain. He said he would park the car and be right in. I went through the whole store doing my shopping. When I got to the checkout line, he still wasn't anywhere to be found. I figured he had run into one of his friends and was busy gabbing.

No, not Jeff, when I went out to find him I saw an ambulance in the parking lot. Naturally I started to panic, especially to see it parked by our station wagon. A lady had fallen, so Jeff had stopped to help her. He soon found out that she was more injured than he had thought at first. He sent someone to call for an ambulance and stuck around helping until the ambulance crew had her loaded up, comforting her all the while. I guess I shouldn't complain at a time in our country where apathy is more the norm. But sometimes I wish he were just a little less friendly. Don't worry, it will never happen; Jeff has too much compassion for mankind.

The afternoon brought with it two things. One was my brother and the second was more chemotherapy. My brother came with his fiancée to see me. My brother, I believe has never dealt with the fact that our other brother died when we were young. He was with him that day and I don't think he ever forgave himself for the accident. I wonder if he carries around the guilt like I do. At least that is my interpretation, I could be wrong.

Now, his sister was living with cancer. He came to see me, because I think he was afraid I was going to die. I could see that in his eyes that day as he came into my room, with fear on his face. After I was diagnosed with leukemia I felt more in tune to people. The look of pity on their faces as they were trying to hold back the fears they themselves were living with. When someone close to you is given bad news you suddenly come face to face with your own mortality.

"Hi!" my brother said as they entered my room.

"I am glad to see you both," I told them. They were the typical yuppie couple of the 1980s. His fiancée was at times a typical blonde. She came from a comfortably wealthy background and was the baby in the family. She was soon to be an addition to the family, this tall, blonde blue-eyed thing with a Barbie-like figure. I was sure envious of her. Do you get the picture? Real live Barbie and Ken dolls.

My brother was always the cute guy, the one that my girlfriends in high school lusted after. He had jet-black hair, and deep brown eyes and olive toned skin. He went on to school and obtained a degree in communications. He is meticulous in all aspects of his life, to the degree that I'm sure he even has the spaces measured in his closet to a half of an inch between each hanger.

Jeff and I were virtually country hicks compared to their circle of friends. We were the homebodies, opposed to the jet set crowd they ran with. Golfing in Arizona in the winter, weekends in New York is the kind of life they lead. While we choose to have popcorn and milk shakes in bed watching TV on a Sunday evening with the children.

Some may say that I was jealous of them. In a way I used to be. I am not anymore. I often envied their freedom and the money they had. But, to be honest with you one of the lessons I learned from my bout with cancer is the importance or shall I say the lack of importance material possessions truly have in life. The amount of money that someone has does not necessarily mean they are happy. We are comfortable, and believe me we are happy. I can't speak for my brother and his wife, I can only speak to what I observe, and I will say that I wouldn't trade my life for theirs any day of the week. I honestly believe I am the freer one in the group.

"You look like you are doing okay," he said, with a relieved tone in his voice, one that kind of made him happy to see I hadn't bought the big one yet.

"I am okay, I've had chemotherapy for almost twenty-four hours and haven't puked yet. I guess that's considered okay," I said, that was enough of an icebreaker to relax us all, after that we all just laughed.

We talked and talked away the afternoon. It seemed to whiz past us with the speed of light. I don't think I have ever felt closer to my brother and soon-to-be sister-in-law as I did that afternoon. The nurse brought in my chemotherapy bag so they all decided that this would be a good time to go and get something to eat. I would be getting some more pre-medication anyway and would more than likely sleep for a while. I watched them leave my room and envied their freedom, to be able to go out to get something eat would've been great, I thought to myself as I drifted off to slumber land.

I slept the entire time they were away. When they returned they brought with them a video to watch, *Johnny Dangerously*. They also had a bag of popcorn. We watched the movie in the early evening and laughed for the entire two hours. That has to be the best medicine I could have ever had.

I was sorry to see them leave when it was time for them to go. They had the long drive back to Minneapolis that night, so they thought they had better get going. They promised they would return the next time they were both in town. His fiancée said that she and her mother might take a drive down to see me one day during the week if they had some time free. I told her that it would be nice to see the both of them again.

The next few days came and went and I kept wondering when I would get sick. You see everyone who had chemotherapy was sick all the time, weren't they? I thought that I was handling this chemotherapy stuff pretty well. At least until later in the week, when suddenly it was like the dam let loose and unleashed a terrible flood of vomit and diarrhea. It was the most disgusting thing I had ever experienced. I never knew that I could throw up that much, let alone so violently.

I have never been one to enjoy vomiting; I swear I could never have become a bulimic because I hate to vomit. There seemed to be no end. The antiemetics they gave me helped some, but not totally, just as they warned me. The waves of nausea came continuously like the waves in the sea. I seemed to be sick all the time, before meals, during meals and when the meal trays were taken away, it was constant. My body was trying to rid itself of these poisons they had dumped into me. Now it decided to help me, where had it been in the battle of not acquiring the disease to start with?

Finally after a week, when the chemotherapy was finished, and so was the nausea, vomiting and diarrhea. All I was left with was weakness. I could barely find the strength to climb in and out of bed. We were waiting now for my white blood cell count to hit rock bottom. That would indicate to them that the chemotherapy had destroyed the cancerous cells that were running rampant in my bone marrow and my body. It would take another week before I would reach that low level; everything was just status quo during that time. Or as status quo it could be under the circumstances.

Chapter Thirteen

I WAS ASSIGNED TO A NEW resident. It had already been long enough, that there was a changing of the guards so to speak. The new one I got I didn't care for at all. The job I had at home gave me plenty of opportunity to work with residents. There are good ones and bad ones.

This one I fondly referred to as the Nazi. I am not really sure where he was from, but he did have a German-sounding accent. Ergo the nickname Nazi, I swear he hated me. He lost me right from the get-go. No sense of humor!

Every time we talked I ended up getting ticked off. Part of the problem I guess was that he never listened to what I said, so why should I try to talk to him? When he would come around in the morning ahead of the rest of the *Dog and Pony Show*, I would often play possum pretending to be asleep. Our daughter when she was little would hide behind a curtain at her grandmother' house and yell, "Can't see me now!" Maybe that is why I pretended to be asleep, so he couldn't see me now.

The *Dog and Pony Show* was the term I used for the grand rounds made every morning. (I can't take all the credit though; it was my sister who came up with it.) First you have the Fellow or Staff physicians, followed by the First or Chief Resident, and finally came all the little residents. Each was being assigned to their own patients, who they would do the ordering of treatments, etc. Naturally, nothing that really could amount to anything would be ordered without the okay of the First. But it reminded me of an act in the circus, the trained lion act where everyone performed in a row all doing the biding of the trainer that carried the whip.

Where if one of them touched me on the shoulder they all touched me on the shoulder, it made me laugh. You know in the old Vaudeville routines where the comedian would somehow glue his shoes to the floor, he then could lean as far as he wanted one way or the other and never fall over. That is just how they were. They would enter the room in a cluster behind the Fellow and the First and lean to the left and lean to the right just like a bunch of trained seals. If the Fellow leaned over to look at something so did they, it was great. That's entertainment! I hope you can get the picture from this or maybe this is one of those things when you had to be there. I laughed up to the time that I developed a rectal abscess, and then I had nine physicians looking up my bottom. This wasn't so funny!

The Nazi and I would never get along. So when they wanted to do a spinal tap on me to see if the leukemia cells had crossed into the cerebrospinal fluid, he wanted to do it. "Not on your life!" I told him. If he wanted to practice, he could go down to the morgue and do it on cadavers, but not on me. If there had been cancer cells in the spinal fluid, it would mean I needed to have chemotherapy injected into the spinal column to treat it.

I was surprised to discover that the same chemotherapy medication they used to destroy the cancer in my bone marrow would not treat cancer in the spinal column. I was afraid of having a spinal tap. I knew the delicate maneuver it was to do one, the only people I knew that did it routinely was someone from the anesthesia department. My resident had decided he would try and talk me into letting him perform mine. NO WAY!

I thought. He could talk until he was blue in the face. There wasn't any way I was going to allow him to stick anything in my body, at anytime or any place.

It was decided that the First/Chief Resident would do it. By this time the job of First/Chief had been transferred to another third year resident. She was different from my friend in that she was more aware of her appearance. She wore makeup, had a stylish haircut and even wore color in her attire. She was slim and had somewhat of a southern drawl to her speech. On our first meeting she said she was told all about me from the other doctors on my case, and that I must be pretty special for them to tell her to take good care of me. I admitted that I was special, because I would get this thing whipped and not even missing a beat out of my life at all. I told her that I would be out of there in as little of time as possible and that I would be cured. Such confidence I boasted with just a few short weeks of treatment under my belt.

I trusted her almost as much as I did the other Chief Resident, she didn't have the same bedside manner, but in her own way I knew she cared. I couldn't imagine her spending hours in the dark talking with me, but she did have a gentleness that allowed me to like her. I really gained a lot of respect for her when she told the Nazi he wouldn't perform the spinal tap under any circumstances. This only made our strained relationship even worse. It was probably good that he only had to spend two weeks with me.

We all have the right to refuse any kind of treatment that we are uncomfortable with and believe me having him perform a spinal tap on me made me more than uncomfortable; it made me break into a cold sweat at the thought of it. I can tell you one thing for sure; he was even more distant and stayed away from me more than usual. I hope that he didn't think it broke my heart any by doing that.

The day I was to have the spinal tap Jeff came up to be with me, I knew that I couldn't handle it alone. I had assisted on most of these procedures too many times both in the Navy and recently as an RN, so the thought of having them performed on me made me panic. He arrived in the late morning, after lunch, which was when the doctor told me she would do it.

I could feel my heart racing when she came into the room. "Are you ready, Jeanine?" she asked. Ready, I thought, what does she mean? If I say I'm not ready she just won't do it? I was getting this done whether I liked it or not, whether I was ready or not.

"I'm as ready as I will ever be!" I replied. My palms were cold and covered with sweat. Jeff just sat there not saying too much. He wasn't looking forward to this either, he was being strong for me because I asked it of him, to come and hold my hand. But he really didn't want to watch or be there in general. He would have done anything for me during this time.

I don't know how he didn't just lose his mind, or up and leave. When a spouse is diagnosed with cancer or any other disease, the family doesn't always survive. It doesn't mean that suddenly they no longer love each other; it is just that they haven't dealt with their own fears concerning life. Not Jeff, he was the only rock in the entire picture. He really believed the part of our wedding vows where it says, "*For better or worse…in sickness and in health, till death do us part.*"

"I told the nurse to give you some pre-medication for this, to help you relax." I sighed after she said that. Immediately after I did, I looked over at Jeff to see if he would chastise me for sighing, but he was preoccupied with the goings-on.

The nurse came in and injected some medication through my Hickman and again the warm rush ran through my body. I could feel myself go almost limp. They draped me across the bedside table and asked me to hunch over. Jeff sat in front of me holding my arms and talking to me. At least there he didn't have to watch them put the needle in. She gave me some lidocaine to numb the area first and finally the spinal needle itself was inserted. I could feel a great pressure in my back and in my legs. Naturally she had great difficulty doing the procedure, I couldn't have a spine that was easily accessible, could I?

I remembered back to the time when they tried to do an epidural block to do a caesarian section on me when I was about to deliver our daughter Jennifer. It didn't work then and they finally ended up giving me a general anesthetic. When they started to make their incision I felt the whole thing. So, of course I would have trouble with a spinal tap too. She told the nurse to give me more medication because I was starting to hyperventilate. That time I really relaxed. I almost went to sleep. After almost thirty minutes she was able to get it. I was so high on the drugs they gave me I just smiled and nodded as I drifted off to sleep.

I woke about an hour later. Jeff was just sitting there watching the television, something he did a lot while waiting for me to wake up from a nap. "I was beginning to think you were out for the night," he said. "That is the worst I've seen. I never knew anyone to have so much trouble." Remember Jeff was a corpsman in the Navy and had assisted with spinal taps just as much as I had, if not more. He had worked in the intensive care unit through most of his stay in Philadelphia. So, he was accustomed to this, but he said it was a lot worse now than back then.

"Did she finally get it?" I asked.

"Yes, but she ended up getting more needles and you more medication. That's why you fell asleep so fast. I thought if she wouldn't have gotten it soon we were going to have to medicate her. She really got upset about not getting it," he said almost laughing.

"That's why I wouldn't let the Nazi do it, could you imagine if he had tried?" I said.

He got up to leave and I asked him, "Where are you going?"

"I have to go home, remember the kids?" he said.

"You can't stay a little while?" I pleaded.

"Jeanine, I have been here most of the day, I can't help it that you slept, but I have to go now. I'll be back this weekend," he said. "I'll have your project for you to start on then too. It'll be about time you start on it, remember what the doctor said? That he wouldn't let you go home until you finished a project. It's already been two weeks. Perhaps you won't get so homesick if you have something to keep your mind busy. He's pretty smart that way, he knows anybody would have a hard time being cooped up in this place, and having you make a project to keep you occupied is a good idea." With that he chuckled.

"Yeah, I guess you are right." I still hated to see him go, it was good to have familiar company. A project would be good to have to do. I had gotten books and magazines, stuff like that, but I still got bored easy. So, the thought of doing a cross-stitch picture sounded like a great idea. A woman who Jeff worked with had sent up a few patterns with him, telling him that once I chose the pattern I liked, she would then go and get the cloth and the thread I would need to complete it. I thought that was quite generous of her to do. It would save Jeff from going and trying to figure the pattern out for himself. I had chosen the saying "Footprints." It had seashells, water, and seagulls in the borders and the rest was words. It would take me the entire time I was there, but I did complete it before I left.

I walked Jeff to the door and gave him a hug good-bye, I told him that I would walk him out to the double doors that cradled the entry to the unit, I should be out walking anyway, I thought. The nurse's station was in the center and the rooms of the unit were like spokes on a bicycle that came out from the circle. So, my walk was around in a circle, like a racetrack of sorts. It was a time that I could walk again free of the pain I had experienced while I was getting the chemotherapy. I was to wear a mask though when I left my room as my white blood cell count was very low. The normal range is 5.5 to 11.0 and mine was .100, which meant I was susceptible to any infection that happened to come along.

Chapter Fourteen

THE WEEKEND BROUGHT JEFF BACK TO me again. It also brought more hair loss. My God it was falling out in clumps. I would pick my head up off my pillow and turn to find more hair on the pillow than on my head. That perhaps was the worst insult of all, total hair loss. Not only my head was bald, but my legs, arms, eyebrows, eyelashes and pubic hair. All gone, even the hair in my nose was gone; it made me feel like an alien of some kind. I was a Bare Naked Lady before those guys made it a popular singing group.

My doctor crashed into the room in his usual whirlwind style. Saturday morning with the rest of the pony show in tow. He took one look at the thinning of my hair and said, "You know that you can continue to lose your hair one by one or you can have the nurses shave it off and be done with it. You see it will all be gone soon. This shaving we find is more comfortable for patients."

He could see by my expression I didn't like the idea too much. "You think about it." With that he left the room in as much of a flurry as he entered. A little like the Tasmanian devil.

"He might be right," Jeff said.

"You mean, have them shave my hair off?" I asked.

"Gig, it's almost gone now. You lose it in big piles. This would make it a little easier maybe...I don't know it was just a suggestion." He shrugged his shoulders.

"It's easy for you to say, you're not the one that will be bald. I hate to make it go any faster. But I will think about it, I promise. Maybe you should bring me back a stocking cap or something," I told him. He gave me a funny look after I said that. "You know to cover my head up when it's gone," I said, pointing to the top of my head.

"What for?" he asked.

"Do you honestly think I'm going to lay here with my head uncovered?" I shouted at him.

"Hey don't bite my head off, I was just asking. I didn't come up here to get yelled at."

"I'm sorry, I didn't mean it." I started to cry. "It's so hard, you know? The chemotherapy, the waiting, the losing of my hair."

He came over and sat on the bed, putting his arms around me. He told me that he would get anything I needed, just tell him what it was. The rest of Saturday went by as usual watching TV, taking naps, holding hands and cross-stitching. Jeff didn't cross-stitch so he took my embroidery floss and wound it around cardboard bobbins. He did this to keep from getting too awfully bored; I don't think he knew just what a big help it was. After he wound as many as he could, he left to head for home. He was driving back and forth so he could spend time in both places, with the children and with me. I felt sorry for him.

We don't realize what a toll an illness takes on the entire family, especially the spouse. We always think of the person with the disease, forgetting the loved ones. These unsung heroes suffer silently. I often think that Jeff needs to write his story, from a caregiver's point of view. In any case the family has to endure quite a bit. Living in a constant state of limbo has to be nerve-racking.

When he left I walked into to the bathroom looking at the hair that remained on my head. I lowered it for a moment and counted about twenty hairs that fell in the sink from the simple movement of bowing my head. It was obvious now that I had to get my hair shaved off. I rang for the nurse.

"Whose the barber? I want you to cut off my hair," I said, as the nurse entered my room.

"Sure, I'm no barber but I guess it's not the style you are looking for, is it?" she quipped.

We decided that I would wait until the next day; she would be here then too. But that way I would have my stocking cap and perhaps a few scarves if I were lucky. After she left the room I called my mother, who was as I said still living with us.

"Has Jeff gotten home yet?" I asked.

"Yes, do you want to talk to him?" she responded.

"Yes, in a minute, but I want you to go and get me some *babushkas* (scarves). I also need a stocking cap. I'm getting my hair cut off tomorrow." Silence for a second or two then I continued, "I'm sure that my little head will get cold without one." I could hear her sigh when I mentioned the fact I would be losing my hair. Even she seemed to have a hard time thinking about it.

"You want some wild ones, it would probably be hard to find a stocking cap to wear this time of year, but we'll see what we can do," she said, and put Jeff on the line.

"What did you call for? Is everything okay?" he asked.

"I wanted to have her pick me out some scarves and stuff. I decided that I would have my hair cut off tomorrow. So bring up the things she picks up, okay?" I asked him.

"I could have bought them, I could have gotten some for you." I could tell that my calling my mother instead of him irritated him. I kind of felt a chill run down my spine; I wished that they could get along for just a few minutes. I'm sure they blamed each other for the fact that I was lying in a bed in Rochester with leukemia. They couldn't see beyond their own noses. Part of the reason I was there was that my loyalties were divided between the two of them. They tried to force me to make choices between them. I didn't know why they couldn't grow closer and support each other instead of breeding the hostilities

111

I knew they harbored towards each other. To be honest with you, looking back on it, I blame the both of them. I needed them both in their own way to help me through this. I refused to argue with Jeff over the fact that I asked my mother to buy the scarves or the hats for me. They were adults and needed to start acting like it.

"I realize that, but I asked her," I told him, refusing to discuss it any further. "How are the kids? Can I talk to them?" That seemed to diffuse the conversation at least momentarily. They both asked me how I was feeling and when I was coming home. I couldn't answer their questions because I didn't know the answers.

I felt a lot of sorrow following the conversation with them. It hurt so much not being able to be there to help them, to hold them. It also angered me some, Jeff and my mother being able to be there. I was jealous of the fact that they were there and I was here. Or was it resentment, I had terribly strong feelings perhaps in both directions. When I finished talking to them I hung up and just sat there for a while.

I went to the closet and got out the bag of cross-stitch supplies Jeff brought me that morning. It was awfully nice of his co-worker to go ahead and get these things for me. I taped the sides of the Aida cloth like I always did with all the cross-stitch projects I have. I then proceeded to find the center of my piece of fabric. It was a beige color; I had never worked on anything but ecru or white cloth before. I wasn't sure if I would like it done in a colored cloth, but I didn't have much choice; it wasn't as if I could run out to the craft store and change it. When I was finished I was happy it was beige.

I soon found the middle and started to count my stitches when I discovered that I would be starting out with the words. The nurse I had that night was doing the same cross-stitch project I was. I called her in and asked her what I should do. She told me that she had started at the top of the project and worked her way down, leaving about a two to three inch border from the top and the sides to have the area to frame the piece when it was completed.

I took her advice and did just that, I counted down and over then started stitching as the project called for and started off making seashells. It was great; I couldn't believe how beautiful it was going to be. I can't believe I doubted the color choice at first. Not anymore, I couldn't seem to put it down once I started it.

The next morning was Sunday; my doctor blew through the door early in the morning with the pony show trotting behind. "As soon as your counts come up we will get another bone marrow biopsy to see how clear the marrow is. If it has less than five percent blasts then you will not need another round of chemotherapy."

"It will be less than five percent," I assured him.

The bone marrow is where the blood cells are produced and there are always a certain percentage of blasts or immature cells in the marrow. The good doctor was telling me that there must be less than five percent of these blast cells in my marrow or I would have to go another round of chemotherapy. I decided that I would be the exception to the rule and have to only have one round of chemotherapy. He told me that very few people ever get away with just one round of chemotherapy; he would hold no promises for me.

Jeff returned around ten in the morning and I told him what the doctor told me. "Jeanine, you must be prepared that you will more than likely have to have another round of chemotherapy. Don't set yourself up to be disappointed." If it was going to be decided on determination alone I know that I would have won that, because I was very determined by this time.

"I just know that I will be the one that doesn't have to go through this again. I just know it." I sighed with that, he knew to not pursue the issue any further with me because I had my mind made up. And once I have made up my mind I don't change it very often.

"Have you started on your project?" he asked, moving on to another subject, he knew it was time to just let me go, even if I was halfcocked. He always sat back just waiting to pick up the pieces whenever I fell apart. I was stubborn and pigheaded.

"Yes." With that I pulled the piece of cloth from the bag it was stored in and showed him the beginning of the project. He watched me work diligently on the sampler the rest of the morning while he wound the many colors of floss he hadn't finished winding the day before. The cardboard bobbins fit neatly in a plastic floss caddy.

Jeff always helped me with projects. How funny it is though because I am so good at starting projects, but not very good at finishing them. I have in our married life started many things; I must have boxes in the basement full of started or half-finished projects. This infuriates him to no end that I say I will make this or that, get all the supplies and never finish it.

My aunt tells me that these are not unfinished projects, I am just preparing for retirement. When on a fixed income I won't be as free to buy my supplies so I am saving up now. I like her explanation better than any I would find in any psychiatric nursing journal I own. It doesn't bother me, I thought, so why should it bother him. I am like this and I have been like this most of my life. I hardly think that his yelling at me now would change me.

The difference is that I was going to finish this project, why was this so different? I had the one big factor in my life that would drive me to the end. My doctor has told me that I would not leave this hospital until I completed My Project! Ha, you think, he can't keep you for a lame excuse like that. Well you have never met my doctor; I know that this man would have arranged it somehow. I wasn't taking any chances; I would complete it before I left.

As I was saying Jeff helps me a lot with my projects, even though he figures they will all end up in the same place, the box in the basement where all good projects go. Besides, what else was there for him to do sitting in a hospital room bored beyond belief, you'd think anything was fun to do just for the distraction.

As Jeff left that night I held on to him tight. Oh, how I wanted to go with him. As the weeks rolled on, the weekends were what I lived for. It was all becoming routine. And when Sunday nights arrived and he would be ready to leave, it grew harder and harder for me to let him go.

It was hard to believe that I could grow to form a routine being in the hospital, but I did. I had my daily blood draws, morning rounds, working on my project, writing letters and watching my favorite soap operas. Some people say they would give anything to just be able to lie around, watch TV and do cross-stitch or some other project, believe me I tell them they do not know what they are saying. I often thought it would be fun too, until the time when thoughts turned to reality. It's like, be careful what you wish for kind of thing.

Chapter Fifteen

WHEN THE WEEKENDS CAME I WOULD be almost on a high from having my husband with me. They say absence makes the heart grow fonder, well in this instance it is true. I was falling in love with Jeff all over again; in this terrible situation I was discovering what about this man I married made me love him in the first place.

You come to a place in any relationship where it can become almost like a comfortable pair of shoes. And you begin, not intentionally mind you, to take the other person for granted. You think that he or she is always there and because of this you become relaxed. You begin to find things that perhaps excite you, it could be your job, your friends, shopping and some have even turned to other relationships.

No don't think that now I am writing a true confessions story, because I am not. I did not turn to someone else and have a sordid love affair, sorry if I disappoint anyone. I realize that I cannot speak for my husband but I think we both feel the same way on this topic, we feel that once married always married. My love for my husband has grown to such depths I cannot even begin to describe it here on paper. If it was my illness that brought me to this point then I thank God for my illness.

Being alone in a hospital with only strangers in your midst gives you plenty of time to reflect on your life. I did that time and time again, I looked back over every inch of my life examining it to see where I may have gone wrong, or at least that is what I thought that I was doing.

After Jeff left, my nurse came into my room with a pair of scissors in her hand. "Your barber has arrived," she said.

"What?" I asked.

"I'm here to cut your hair, I waited until Jeff left before I came in. I didn't think that you wanted him to be here when I did it so I waited. You haven't changed your mind, have you?" she asked.

"No, I guess I just forgot about it. No, I haven't changed my mind. Let's get it over with." I walked over and sat in a chair next to my bed.

I looked into the bag that Jeff brought with him containing the stocking cap and some scarves he and my mother bought for me. In there were a couple of nice silky scarves, some bandanas, and a bright red stocking cap. My God, I thought, bright red! I didn't particularly want to resemble a stoplight; I just wanted to keep my silly head warm.

She started with the scissors and just cut my hair to about a half an inch in length all over my head. I looked like a refugee from a holocaust camp. In fact, I told her if she knew of any auditions for parts in a movie about the holocaust I would be free soon. We laughed, and when she left my room I went into the bathroom and looked in the mirror. Once again all I could do was cry. It didn't take very long to cut my once golden tresses to their new length. I thought to myself that Jeff probably hadn't even gotten out of the city yet and I was bald…

That next week came and at the end of it my counts finally reached a point that they scheduled a bone marrow biopsy for that Friday. The thought of this made me start to shake, I hate those things, and they are almost unbearable. Jeff wouldn't be able to get away for this one either.

His job was beginning to give him some difficulty each time he left early. He also was working most every Saturday before this happened. He was no longer able to do that so they told him he would have to take vacation days to make up the time. At a time when this man was hitting the lowest point in his life, the potential loss of his wife, the life he was used to. The life he had become comfortable with.

And now they would hassle him about wanting to be with me, I only prayed they never had to face a similar situation. I sometimes think that compassion has totally gone out of the picture when it comes to business. My husband worked with a gal who also had leukemia and they took away her job because she wasn't able to be at work. It was policy that after six months you no longer had a job. She eventually lost her life...I say screw the job, take care of you first.

You spend a good majority of your life in a job and with the people you work with. Perhaps you spend more time with the people you work with than you spend with your own family. And that is not how you handle someone who has given you ten years of loyal work. To tell a man who has been devastated by his wife's illness, trying to hold a family together, he would have to use his vacation to cover the time not spent on weekends was a very cruel thing to do in my opinion. In fact, it was the most unforgivable thing I have ever heard of. Time heals all wounds though and I guess I understand the concept even if I don't understand the lack of compassion. The old adage "the show must go on," right?

The next morning I woke early so I could shower and dress before my bone marrow. It was kind of like preparing the "vestal virgin" for sacrifice. (You couldn't get the dressings wet after the bone marrow biopsy.) I felt as if I was being prepared for the sacrificial volcano, instead for me it was a sacrificial bone marrow.

Or should I be honest and say that I didn't ever really sleep well the night before I was to have a bone marrow test done. I waited almost till eight o'clock before they showed up to do it. They were standing outside of my door. I could feel my heart race; the adrenaline was pulsing through my body. My nurse went to get the pre-medication that the doctor had ordered for me to have, and began injecting it through my Hickman catheter. I could feel the medication effects come over me. It seemed like it started at the core of my being and continued rushing through my entire body. I started to relax.

Earlier that morning while I was getting dressed my nurse came in and told me all about one of the RNs who does bone marrows, her name was Mae. She was supposed to be one of the best ones. She didn't know this from personal experience mind you, but from the stories the other patients told her. Not that the other RNs who performed them weren't good, but she was supposed to be exceptional. I asked, "How do I get Mae, can I request her?" She was supposed to be so good that you barely felt any pain and I knew at that moment she was the gal for me.

"No, she takes her turn on the hospital rotation like all the others, so if she's on you'll have her. There is this guy down the hall that will do just about anything to get Mae to do his bone marrow. He's down there now praying for her to be the one." With that she laughed. "There was a time he told me that when he was supposed to have a bone marrow in the clinic, he even told them he was one of Mae's relatives, thinking that would get him preferential treatment." She really laughed this time and then exited the room.

She thinks this is funny! I'd do just about anything too, I thought, I'll even pray to have her right then, and I did. But it was to no avail, it wasn't Mae who walked into my room that morning it was the same woman who had been doing the bone marrows in the clinic the day I had my first one. She told me that Mae was doing the procedures in the clinic now and that she was on the hospital service. What luck I thought!

I was starting to feel groggy from the medications they had given me. As I drifted into a semiconscious state I thought to myself if I can't have Mae then at least I'll do the drug thing. In fact, I became quite sleepy, and even though the pain was just as intense as before, somehow this time it was more tolerable.

I drifted off to sleep after they were finished. I slept for nearly two hours. When I awoke from my drug-induced nap, I had the same painful feeling in my hip that I remembered from before. I was happy it was only one hip this time that was at least in my favor. All I could hope for is that if I had to have any more I was going to pray it would be this Mae person doing it.

Now, the real waiting began. It wouldn't be until the next morning that I would be told the results of the bone marrow biopsy. I just waited patiently, hoping for the best. Believe me I wasn't as calm as I am making it sound here. I was a nervous wreck! I told everyone that I would be one of the ones that would need only one round of treatment but deep in my heart I was afraid I was wrong. My husband kept trying to prepare me for the disappointment and as usual I refused to listen to him.

The next morning while Jeff and I watched TV the doctor rolled in. His face not as bright as it usually was. "Mrs. Marster, we will have to do another round of the chemotherapy. You are not in remission where I would like you to be. The treatment will begin tonight, so be prepared. You must continue to work on the project, you cannot go home until it is finished." Why? I couldn't believe my ears. I could feel Jeff's arm on my shoulder as I was trying to fight back the tears.

"Was my marrow still full of the leukemia cells?" I asked.

"There were eight percent blast cells in the marrow," he told me.

"Eight percent, for a lousy three percent I am going to have more chemotherapy? That's not fair!" I told him. I am now being haunted by my own words to my children. Don't you just hate that? I always tell them that there are a lot of things in life that are not fair. Well I have myself now met one of them. I must remember to apologize to them forever using that phrase.

I remember in the movie *The Agony and the Ecstasy* Charlton Heston played Michelangelo, and Rex Harrison played the Pope. It was when the Pope commissioned Michelangelo, to paint the Sistine Chapel. In the movie it showed that during the many year project Michelangelo would oftentimes be disruptive during mass.

120

The Pope always looked up at him on the scaffold and mouthed the words, "When will you be through?" This always came about after some paint had fallen on his robe, or a piece of scaffolding fell.

Michelangelo would simply reply while he was painting, stopping only briefly to check out where the stuff landed. "When I am finished," he mouthed back at him. There would always be this stalemate between the two of them for what seemed to last forever.

Now I am not saying that the project I was creating was a masterpiece, but every time he asked me about completing my project I would simply answer him, "When I am finished," smiling back at him.

He left the room so fast that I couldn't give him a hard time for making me have more chemotherapy. He knew better than to stand around here too long, I would have given him a severe tongue-lashing. He is getting to know me!

My God, I failed! What was I going to do? More chemotherapy more sickness, more time away from my husband and children. The one glowing thing that I could hold on to was that I wouldn't get anymore bald.

"It'll be okay," Jeff said as he tried to reassure me that I wasn't the failure I thought I was. Good job, Jeff, why don't you just say I told you so and be done with it? Why did he sound almost relieved by this?

"How can you say that? I have to have more chemotherapy, and it will start tonight! I have to stay here longer! I can't come home!" With that I burst into tears.

Then he said the one thing I had hoped he would refrain from saying. "I tried to warn you that it might not work out the first time." I could have gone the rest of my life, or at least that day, without ever hearing those words. They acted like fingernails on a chalkboard. The hair on the back of my neck started to stand up, which must've been all two of them.

"I know..." was all I could muster up to say. He was right and I couldn't deny it. I always hated it when he was right though.

121

This time was no different. Yet, I knew I had set myself up for this one. I was not preparing for the fact that I may need more chemotherapy.

On the other hand I was using positive thinking to a certain degree. I was positive that I was going to have just one round. And the doctor was positive that I was going to have two, no matter what the tests showed. I believe that the first time he told me some people would have just one round he knew then that I would have to have two. Somewhere in the devious little French mind of his was Michelangelo creating in me his Sistine Chapel and I was the Pope forever wanting it to be finished before it was actually done.

"It won't be so bad. You've already been through this once," Jeff said. Easy for him to say, I thought. He isn't the one that will be sick all the time. Now when I was just starting to get my appetite and strength back. I was losing weight, never having been a skinny Minnie anyway; I had lost another ten pounds in just three weeks. Goodness, three weeks was all I was here, I guess it's true what they say, that time flies when you are having fun. Are we having fun yet?

Appetite loss would continue to plague me each time I would have a treatment of any kind. Subconsciously, I thought if I didn't eat then I wouldn't puke. I was glad I had the extra reserve, overweight, or I might have had the body to go along with the holocaust hair. So, at this time at least plump was perfect!

Chapter Sixteen

Jeff went to Hardee's and got us both chef's salads, when he finally got me as calmed down as he could. For some strange reason I was craving them. He also brought me a milkshake. Wow, for once in our married lives he was actually letting me eat anything I wanted. I know that sounds weird, but you see all the years we've been married I have been overweight. I was constantly asking him to help me lose it. So, he would play warden with every morsel that wasn't supposed to pass through my lips, he would give me the evil eye. Now that I was instructed to eat I was going to take advantage of it, right? That is at least until tomorrow. Jeff spent the weekend at the Holiday Inn down the street. He was able to stay longer with me in the evening. It was great, we didn't do too much but it was the time spent together that meant the most.

The next morning I was hanging my head in the puke bucket when he arrived. Remember I already told you I never liked throwing up and I hated it even more, I also never liked to clean it up. Now, I found myself vomiting much too frequently. This brought in the antiemetics (anti nausea drugs). After this, I would settle down for a while. I guess I was going to be sicker this round than with the first.

Jeff spent the rest of the weekend sitting patiently at my bedside as I drifted in and out of la-la land. A place I would venture off to during most of my chemotherapy. I eventually came out of it when I was through with the medication. He would only leave long enough for his short treks to the Kahler Hotel coffee shop for a cigarette, a cup of coffee and some more conversation with total strangers. People that were trying to find sanity in all of the insanity. The families of those that lay in hospitals undergoing treatments for all kinds of illnesses, needed someone and usually they would find peace at the counter even if for only a moment. It was like group therapy for all of them.

The next few weeks brought with them more low blood counts and lots of high fevers. I hit an all-time high of 40 degrees Celsius or shall I say that in Fahrenheit it was 104 degrees. This is when I knew I reached a point of delirium. I kept telling my friends back home that the nurses were trying to kill me. Wow, was I whacked out or what? Why would they be trying to do that when they were actually trying to save me? The way I felt though, I guess I thought they were trying to do the opposite. Behold the power of the mind!

During a conversation with a friend from home, I mentioned I was craving dill pickles and tomato juice. I shouldn't have been surprised one afternoon when a nurse from home stopped by to see me. She was attending classes in Rochester for her bachelor's degree in nursing and thought she would deliver the things I had requested. Naturally living with modern chemistry, as I was I never remembered making a request for anything.

The dill pickles and tomato juice combination made me throw up promptly once she left my room. Of course it couldn't have had anything to do with the fact that I ate ten pickles and drank two glasses of tomato juice while in her presence. Believe me that it was the combination from hell. I think I would have thrown up even without the effects of the chemotherapy. The mere thought of it now while writing this makes me shudder. I don't think anyone should have listened to me. The drugs had me saying and doing things I really didn't mean.

I couldn't believe the many people I heard from while I was in the hospital. I swear the only thing that kept me sane at times, was mail call. It was in the afternoon and I would generally receive at least two cards or letters every day. I became conditioned to waiting for mail while Jeff spent six months in Okinawa during the first year we were married. Here I was again waiting for the mail to keep me attached to the people I cared about. I started putting the cards up on the walls and the windows of my hospital room. I tried to cover the entire room with them, I must admit thanks to all the people I knew back home I did a fairly good job of redecorating.

I wasn't able to receive real flowers in the BMT unit. It was because of the bacteria and mold that are harbored in the soil of real plants and flowers. That is why they wouldn't let you have them. So, I received many very nice silk flower arrangements. Some of these I still have displayed in my home today. Between the silk flowers and the Mylar balloons I must've kept a flower shop in business.

I can never thank the people enough that spent both their time and money on me. Their thoughtfulness will never be forgotten and will always be appreciated. Because as I said these things were my lifeline that connected me to home. The feeling of isolation didn't help my claustrophobia any; in fact, I think it may have heightened it, so anything that was a diversion was welcomed.

This experience certainly changed my feeling about visitors in the hospital after hours. I allow people who are visitors on the unit I worked at to stay longer because of my stay in the hospital. Contact with people does more for some patients than any shot in the arm I could give them.

I mentioned fevers earlier, well my fevers were spectacular. I was immediately started on antibiotics, strong ones too I might add each time I had a fever spike. Ones that eventually sent my liver enzymes out into orbit. Ones that also caused a fiery red rash on my body that resembled a huge welt. It itched so badly and I was so swollen that I knew now what a lobster might look and feel like. I looked terrible! They seemed very perplexed by it too. No one was sure where it all was coming from. Finally they called it a "drug fever." They stopped everything all at once, so we never really knew which medication caused the reaction.

Speaking of rashes, you know that the rash that sent me to the doctor in the first place, then to this place? The day after my first dose of chemotherapy it disappeared! It was almost like clockwork, I got the chemotherapy and they started to dissolve before my eyes, like magic.

I kept telling them (doctors and nurses) to let me go home, that I was a chemistry major and if they gave me the right formulas. I'm sure I could pour equal amounts of *Janitor in the Drum* and *Drano* from under my kitchen sink. I believe I would have gotten the same results. I could have my Cheerio's in the morning along with toxic waste and I'd be good to go. I had a hard time comprehending the fact that I was actually having poison running through my veins.

Jeff teased me by telling me that when I came home he would get some good mink oil to put on my baldhead. He figured I must glow in the dark from all the chemicals I had. I was too afraid to open my eyes in the dark to see for sure. When there was a full moon he promised he would get a good shine on my head and leave the blinds open on the windows in our bedroom so I could be used as a nightlight. He told me that he wasn't cheep, he would make sure it was the "good" stuff.

I told you about the fevers and low blood counts, not only in my white blood cell counts, but also in my red blood cell counts. I was now getting regular transfusions. I would receive two units whenever my hemoglobin would dip down in the 7 gm range; the normal is 12 to 16 gm. I would turn as white as the sheets that I lay on even with the rash you could see how pale I was. I would get weak and dizzy especially if I made any sudden changes in my position.

During this time was when I really looked sick. I wore the red stocking hat on my head at all times, or scarves, just something to cover up. I had now lost another thirteen pounds. My eyes had these dark circles around them. My nail beds were pale and blue in color. I'm not painting a very pretty picture, am I? I couldn't believe what a difference a little blood could do though, I would actually pink up a little bit after receiving a transfusion, or as I called it topping off my tank. I started to look almost human instead of the holocaust refugee I mentioned earlier.

Chapter Seventeen

WE FINALLY MADE IT THROUGH THE rough spots in the road and my counts were getting better. I started to even feel human again. Jeff decided that after six weeks the kids could come up to see me. I was getting closer to going home. I had survived what we thought was the worst of it and I needed to see the kids as much as they needed to see me. I didn't know how they would react to me. On the one hand I was almost afraid to see them. On the other hand I could hardly wait.

He had to prepare them that I looked different, that I wore scarves instead of hair and I had become very weak. I am sure they were just as afraid as I was. In fact the other day I decided to ask them a few questions about that first time they saw me. It brought back a lot of painful memories for them; Jennifer did finally admit that she was really scared to see me. She wasn't sure what she would find, so coming to see me that first time made her nervous. Justin couldn't remember too much, but he agreed he shared some of those same feelings.

I felt like I needed to get to know them all over again. I didn't realize that even though life was on hold for me, for them life continued to be the same. They went to school every day, did their homework, played with friends, go shopping and to swim meets all without me. I guess I must have wanted them to experience the same limbo that I was experiencing so I didn't miss anything. I felt that I was being left out on so much of them, their lives. How unfair is that? Jeff tried as best he could to make their lives as normal as possible.

The morning they came to see me, I was so excited. Jennifer hung back for a while before she would come up to me. Not Justin, he just flew into my arms. All I could do was cry. My babies, what would I do without them? What would happen to them if I were not there? No, I won't think this way! I will think positively. I will not leave them now or ever. Please God let me stay with them. Let me help you watch over them. You gave them to me to take care of, not to leave them now.

"I miss you, Mom. I miss you a lot. When do you get to come home?" Justin asked. He was the most accepting of me, he seemed to just bounce around as if I hadn't ever left. He never seemed to pay much attention to the fact I wore a scarf on my head. I loved them so much that I could actually feel my heart ache when he asked me that question.

"Soon, Justin, soon," was all I could muster up to say.

"You want Mom to be well when she comes home, don't you?" Jeff helped me out. Justin nodded. "Well, she has to finish her treatments and then she will be home." I nodded at them. Jennifer kept hanging in the background, not really saying too much. Just observing me from a distance. I missed them! I knew I did, I just didn't know how much until that very moment.

"Jennifer, how is school?" I finally broke our silence and asked her.

"Fine." Smiling her little Jennifer smile.

"How is swimming going?" I followed. She had finished earlier in the month and I had forgotten that. I was trying to make small talk with my own daughter. How sad was that?

I had forgotten the big dilemma that had arisen about who would take the kids to the C-Finals swim meet in Cedar Rapids.

Jeff felt that he needed to be with me, he also wanted them to go and participate. Finally, my mother volunteered to take them. I couldn't believe she would do that, but she did. Thanks, Mom!

The weather was bad with snow. Jennifer didn't do very well at the competition, so she wasn't that fun to be with. The ultimate insult came at the end of the meet, when my mother's car broke down three hours from home. She got it running enough to follow some friends of ours back to Mason City, limping along all the way.

Her response brought me back from my thoughts. "We're done until summer session, except for stroke clinic," she replied. Stroke clinic was a time that the swim coaches would take a week to work on one stroke at a time. Seeing as there are four strokes, the clinic lasted four weeks.

She didn't accuse me of being disinterested or dumb for not remembering the big meet. We were all trying too hard to get along. You see, normally Jennifer would have told me I was dumb for forgetting this. But, now Mom was ill and no one wanted to upset me. People would make allowances for me, because I have cancer. I wonder if I was to have robbed a bank if they would have made such allowances for that too. Cancer seemed to make a difference in a lot of things that happened. Everyone walked like they were on eggshells not wanting to stress me out.

The rest of their visit went the same way, except as I said for Justin. He sat on the edge of my bed or sat on my lap for the most part. Jennifer didn't come near me; she spent most of the time in a chair near my bed. Finally, just before she left she warmed up enough to come over and sat with me for a while. In fact, when it was time to leave she didn't want to go.

I could see from my own experiences with tragedy as a child that my daughter was going to grow up too fast and have her childhood robbed from her. That really made me mad at God; you see He is in control of the situation so why did Jennifer and Justin have to suffer?

I was taken out of my own childhood at nine and forced to

live in an adult world. Why couldn't my children have been spared this? I lost my brother and six months later I lost my father. They were accidents but, life changed for my other brother and I in one day. So this cancer thing really made me mad.

On our anniversary March 18, 1989, Jeff took the day off and came to see me. He brought with him two new fluted champagne glasses, whipped cream and a bottle of Asti-Spumante. I had received a basket of fruit as a gift that contained a pint and a half of strawberries. That was what the whipped cream was used for. We celebrated our life together in such a special way that Jeff even today talks about it being one of the best anniversary celebrations ever. I remember it as being bittersweet; bitter because of where we were and sweet because we were together. I lay in bed getting another blood transfusion and Jeff stayed next to me holding my hand from time to time.

Later that afternoon my pastor called and asked me if it would be okay to call me during the service the next morning. He wanted to talk to me about my anger that I felt when I was taken sick. I told him it would be all right to call me. When the next morning arrived I was nervous, to the point of nausea. I am not a public speaker, nor do I profess to be one. I hated to talk to strangers even more. My only salvation through all of this was I didn't have to look anyone in the eyes. I couldn't see them at all. I did pray for guidance for what to say to these people. All I had to do was answer the questions that he asked. I told them how I immediately got angry with God when I learned my diagnosis. I was holding Him responsible for this whole mess.

Later some people that knew my mother and attended our church told her there wasn't a dry eye in the house. I talked to them about priorities, love and anger. They said they all examined their own lives a little by the time I was finished. You see even though I was angry with God I discovered that it was an okay thing to do at times. Perhaps, I was able to help someone alter his or her own course of life by re-prioritizing. I know that I certainly did.

131

The day came when after all the blood draws, blood cultures, antibiotics, transfusions, vomiting, bloody urine and diarrhea, I was going to have another bone marrow biopsy. This time I knew for certain it would be a remission marrow. And I would be done with all this! I knew it because I met Mae and she promised me a good slide. They were right! I was able to better tolerate the pain when Mae performed the bone marrow biopsy. It must have been her soothing voice; it was soft and gentle like a fluffy cloud. Or was it like the power of suggestion? I was absolutely sure it wouldn't hurt if Mae did the biopsy.

Mae wasn't at all what I expected when I met her. She was a short white-haired lady who spoke almost in a whisper. Her smile stretched across her entire face, I'm sure it encompassed the universe. Her eyes glistened with such a twinkle that she reminded me of an elf. She, and the tender loving care she gave me, instantly mesmerized me. Yes, Mae you were my angel. God sent you to me at a time when I was in great despair. You came, reached out your hand and lifted me out of my pit. You are my hero!

My marrow was clean! Houston, we have remission! I was going to go home, but I was to come back in three weeks. That was the next shock of my life; I didn't evidently pay attention at the beginning of all this because I was now being told that I had to come back for two more rounds of chemotherapy. I was puzzled. "Let me get this straight, I am in remission, right? But I have to come back for more chemotherapy? I'm missing something here. Will someone explain it to me?"

"You have to undergo two more rounds of chemotherapy, one in about three weeks, and a third about three weeks after that," the Chief Resident told me.

"Why? What happened? I thought that I would go into remission and that would be it, I would never have to come back again." How wrong I was. You see all protocols are different. The protocol that I was following hits you hard with the chemotherapy all at once. The other protocol had you stretch it out over a period of years for treatment. I was lucky I guess to get it all up front. Even though I knew it was the best idea, I didn't like it.

I was sad that day. I thought I would never have to see this place again. Not that I hadn't been forming some definite attachments to the staff, I simply didn't want to be sick anymore. All I knew at that moment was that I was going to be able to go home. I guess I would deal with the coming back when the time came. At this precise moment I was going to leave! The biggest thrill of my life after eight weeks of being cooped up, I was going home. Hallelujah!

A couple of the nurses who worked the night shift, just before I was ready to go home made me a pair of "designer shorts" as a gift to remember them by. Patients always wore gowns and white shorts in the hospital in Rochester. Back home the patients wore pajama bottoms. All I cared about was having my backside covered. I wasn't going to be exposed any more than I needed to be.

These gals took a pair of shorts along with some fabric pens, making a new kind of fashion statement. It was the most wonderful and touching thing they could have ever done. It was so wonderful that my husband, Jeff, had them framed. We went to a local framer and they made a sort of shadowbox for them. The main focus of the shorts was, the list they made up telling the tale of an average day in the life of a leukemic. Here it is:

Average Day in the life of a Leukemic

1 a.m.	Puke
2 a.m.	Heavy Doses of Ativan/Compazine/Benadryl
3 - 4 a.m.	Ozone Layer
5 a.m.	Blood Draw
6 a.m.	Resident (Nazi) Exam
7 a.m.	Shift Change: Exit Crabby Night Nurse
8 a.m.	Breakfast Tray - Increased Nausea
9 a.m.	Shower
10 a.m.	Dog and Pony Show
11 a.m.	Site Care

12 p.m.	Lunch Tray - More Nausea
12 - 3 p.m.	Blood Transfusions
3 to 4 p.m.	Hives/High Temperature - Enter Resident (Nazi)
5 p.m.	Blood Cultures
6 p.m.	Supper Tray - Nausea
7 p.m.	Exit Crabby Day Nurse
8:01 - 8:08 p.m.	Feel Good
9 p.m.	Ampho Rigors
10 p.m.	Dose of Demerol
11 p.m.	Puke
Midnight	Chemo Finally Here
Repeat Day	Times 3 Weeks

The day I left I couldn't believe how much stuff I had accumulated and needed to pack. I was exhausted just getting it all organized. I couldn't believe how weak I was. I tired easily. I got up that morning early. I was working on getting it all together so that when Jeff got there he could take me home. I would be ready to go. He arrived late morning, by lunchtime I was being wheeled out of the unit by the hospital escort; with my complete project in hand.

I was not used to being in shoes. For these two months, my feet were used to being in socks only, that's all I wore in the hospital. Now, I was trying to squish them into sneakers and they strongly objected.

When we got to the front door of the hospital, I was amazed at how loud things were outside. Not being able to go out of my room for two months made me very sensitive to the outdoor noises. The traffic was almost deafening. The smells were very intense also. It was definitely a type of sensory overload. Even though the noises and the smells gave me somewhat of a headache, I was glad to be free. I can't imagine how intense it must be for someone coming out of prison after many years because it was overwhelming for me just coming out of the hospital after two months.

The ride home had me looking at everything quite intensely. I guess I had never truly looked at the sky, the trees and the grass or farmers fields before. It all seemed so different now; I didn't want to miss anything. I was soaking it all in like a sponge. *Never again*, I told myself, would I let this earth just pass by me like it had before. I wanted to take it all in, savoring every intoxicating breath.

We got to a remote part of the countryside, with only a farmhouse off in the distance and many miles of fields around us. It was there I asked Jeff to pull the car over. The Mylar balloons I received while in the hospital were going to be set free. I realize that it isn't good for the environment but to me it was a symbol of freedom, my freedom. As I watched them soar up in the sky, I felt like I was the one being set free and I wanted to soar right alongside them...

Chapter Eighteen

WHEN WE PULLED INTO THE DRIVEWAY that day, there was a banner strung across the garage door that read, "Welcome Home Mom." The kids had gotten their babysitter to print off of her computer a banner for them to color; they even remembered to stay in the lines. There are two maple trees that sit in front of our house on the parking; they were tied with yellow ribbons. Granny had told them about the Tony Orlando and Dawn hit song from the seventies "Tie a Yellow Ribbon Round the Old Oak Tree." They had no clue what it all meant but I sure did. So when I saw their gesture of love I smiled and then cried. It is difficult at times to be female, always crying at the drop of a hat. I never knew why we as women do that but it seems to always come down to tears.

The tension between Jeff and my mother hadn't improved much over the time I was hospitalized. In fact, it may have increased a bit. Especially when Jeff asked her to move out. Why now? Why not the night she stopped by, I thought to myself. I wouldn't have made myself sick stressing over the two of them. At least that is how I saw things. I was always trying desperately to please everyone.

It was actually not so bold as it sounds; Jeff honestly misunderstood the discharge rules I was given. He thought we had to get rid of the dogs, cats, plants and the like, all for my protection. So, because she had a dog and two cats herself he thought that this would be an opportunity for her to go out on her own. After all, it had now been eight months. It was time to leave the nest so to speak.

It wasn't until we actually left the hospital we found out that the restrictions we received weren't exactly meant for me. These were the restrictions they placed on bone marrow transplant patients. By this time there had been enough hard feelings between the two of them that he left it at that, letting her move out.

She made arrangements to move into half of the duplex she owned just down the street from us. The duplex was part of her divorce settlement. She could live in one half while renting out the other half. It was like going home for her anyway; this is the same place she and my stepfather lived when they first moved to Iowa.

She was already comfortable living there. She still knew most of the neighbors. It was also where Jennifer, Jeff and I lived after Justin was born. It would now be a source of income for her. I realize that it wasn't what she wanted to do but it was for the best. I had lived under the same roof with my mother and husband for eight months and they were the worst eight months of my life. I couldn't handle the stress any longer!

I don't want anyone to get the wrong idea. I love my mother dearly. But, I am also not always comfortable with her. I suppose after all the things I grew up with and when she had her accident, I was just as reserved in our relationship as Jennifer was with me that first time we saw each other while I was still in the hospital. I remembered when I saw my mother in a wheelchair the first time after her car accident, I was terrified. On the one hand, I wanted to run into her arms and have her take all the pain I felt away. On the other hand, I was also angry with her for messing up my life the way she did. Sounds selfish, doesn't it?

It's hard when you are young to figure things out. For Jennifer at age eleven only knew nothing other than how to be a child. Suddenly she was faced with much more, and I was the one person who had done this to her. How could she not be angry with me? I would expect no less from either of my children because I was mad at me too. Just as I was mad at my mother back when my brother and father died and she had her accident. The only difference is that I have discussed the anger with my children; I never did with my mother.

Anger eventually turns to resentment if allowed to fester. I believe this was what happened to my mothers and my relationship. We are at a point now, where I can say "no" to her even if she gets mad at me she realizes that I still love her. It is okay to disagree, my mother was always used to my agreeing with anything she said. That is why I left home the way I did (running away to Minneapolis to live with my sister) at the age of eighteen. Because, I felt life at home was too hard. Doesn't every eighteen-year-old?

When I walked into our house that first afternoon, Jeff had to corral our dogs. Our collie's name was Keebler, named after the Keebler cookie elves. What else would you name a dog that was born in a hollow tree? Someone that my husband works with came up with the name, so we cannot take full credit for the creativity. She was my baby, so naturally, when she saw me after almost two months she nearly knocked me over showing me affection. She wiggled, squinted her eyes and rolled onto her back crying the entire time. It was as if to say, "Please pet me, Mom, I really missed you." That is the one thing that I thoroughly enjoy about pets is they are truly devoted to you and they love unconditionally.

The other pets were also in among the welcoming party. They consisted of the collie, a miniature schnauzer named Fritz, a Siamese cat named Yin and a mixed breed orange cat named Marmalade. The cats naturally were more standoffish but their being there was enough to let me know of their enthusiasm. Fritz, the old man in the group, just barked and jumped up and down.

I walked around the house very carefully, inspecting every inch of the place. Taking in all the sounds, sights and smells I had desperately longed for. I couldn't believe I was actually home. It was my home and these are my things. I now know how Dorothy felt in the *Wizard of Oz*. I truly believed at that moment in time, there was no place like home. I know that I told everyone where I had been and that I just wanted to go home, just like Dorothy did. Finally, I was sent here and all the people that love me surround me. Thank you, God!

A friend of mine stopped by the house about then and we had a wonderful visit. She was also a coworker. I told her I needed to go visit the rest of my friends (coworkers) at the hospital. I asked if she could take me when she had time. She agreed to take the time to get me up there whenever I was ready to go. I was more than ready. We decided upon the following Tuesday, at shift change to catch as many of the staff we could from the two shifts. I wanted her to go with me for several reasons, the main one being that I didn't want to go up there alone. If she could take me, then Jeff wouldn't need to take more time off work.

I felt that I owed these people at least a visit; they were all so good to me while I was in the hospital. The cards, gifts, flowers, phone calls, the times they brought dinner over to my family while I was away was unbelievable. We often think that in this day and age, is there really anybody that cares anymore? You hear of people being mugged on the streets and no one stopping to help, well my faith in humanity had been restored. There are still people being mugged and people still don't stop. But, there were those there for my family when I couldn't be.

All the way from the teacher my daughter had in the fifth grade that took her to dinner one evening because, she was so upset about my illness. Or the neighbors that brought over dinners. The people my mother and Jeff knew from other businesses that paid for my husband to stay in a hotel one weekend while he came to visit me in Rochester. We didn't know how to say thank you for all they did for us. How could I not have my faith restored in humanity as I said? These people in

Iowa, these friends (coworkers) have given me back the faith that I was searching for.

Isn't it funny, there I was working and living. When suddenly my life was changed in a way I cannot believe, for the rest of my life. I will say that at the time, I didn't know the changes that would take place were some of the best changes ever. I didn't know that out of the rubble of what was my life there has now emerging a more wonderful new life. Did you ever see the movie with Jimmy Stewart in it, *It's a Wonderful Life?* Well, I felt that same jubilation as George did. I guess one must have to have a brush with death to appreciate how fragile life is. As well as how much it has to offer. All you have to do is just hang on for the ride!

Once my friend left I continued to walk around my house taking everything in. I still couldn't believe I was really home. I could actually cook and clean again. Isn't that a laugh! Can you believe I actually could hardly wait to do those things? Before I was ill I complained miserably about having to dust, vacuum and do laundry. Now, like a crazy person, I was actually looking forward to doing them all once again. I couldn't start right then though because I was still too weak. The day's activities to this point had worn me out. I needed to go at things slowly. Take each day one at a time. To this day I always try to push myself to do more, when I should take the time to slow down. I do love being alive!

Well, this is one area that has really changed. I used to be one that hated to be idle, you know the saying that "idle hands are the devil's workshop" well I didn't like to sit still before and now I was much worse. I found that I hated to waste time; we don't know how much time we have left. Each precious day is given to us and we must live it to the fullest. So I was determined or shall I say obsessed to the point of insanity about sitting still. As soon as I regained all my strength I even took on new projects. I believed I was spared death because I was now going to save the world. That is how euphoric I had become about life. I had all the answers, right?

When the children arrived home after school there was more hugging, kissing and laughing. Oh yes, I have learned a house that is full of laughter is a much happier place to come home to. There isn't much anymore that this family doesn't laugh about. I did find that it is hard to discipline your children when they crack you up all the time. I remembered this about my own youth. My brother and I discovered early in life that if we could make Mom laugh then the punishment wasn't as severe.

Life was once again good to us. I had managed to push all of it out of my mind. You don't have to deal with it if you just don't think about it. I always seemed to be able to suppress things that had happened in my life that were too painful to deal with. All of my tragedies were back somewhere in the recesses of my mind. They were waiting to haunt me someday, if I didn't deal with each and every demon. I say demon because, that is how I referred to them when each calamity occurred.

We all have our demons that we choose not to battle. We all like to be a little bit like Scarlet O'Hara dealing with everything tomorrow. Things do tend to look better in the morning, I must admit. The question is that when the tomorrow came did Scarlet ever deal with her problems; do any of us deal with our problems in the dawn's early light? For me anyway, the answer was no and that is why I still battle my demons day by day now.

The cancer demon, perhaps the scariest of all for me, will take a bit longer. All the others don't seem as insurmountable any more. I have identified the demons, but I am not battling them any longer. I have chosen not to challenge them any longer. Why, you might ask? Well I have learned to live in the present and to let the past stay there. I realized that some of the things I have suppressed in my past were gone for a reason. I have obviously forgotten these as a way to protect myself. I find just knowing what they are is enough for me now. Is this survival or is this just another form of avoidance. I don't have a degree in psychology, and won't pursue one. As it comes to me now, who cares?

141

Chapter Nineteen

I HAD ONLY THREE WEEKS AT home with my family before going back to Rochester for another round of chemotherapy. They were three of the most wonderful weeks I had experienced in quite awhile. The first thing I did was use the golf clubs that Jeff had purchased for me the year before. A friend of mine had given me the basics of golf that summer. In fact, it was because of her tutelage that I was given my own set of clubs as a present from Jeff for my birthday, a lady's starter set. I have since been given a full set with metal woods, which was another birthday present from Jeff.

Another friend taught me the rest. She told me that once I had the basics down, club handling, putting, driving and retrieving the ball when out of bounds, all I needed to do was to put it all into practice. I dragged her around more golf courses than anyone would have ever imagined. Remember I told you; I never wanted to sit still. Well that is why we golfed many summer days away. I remember the laughter we shared, as well as the warm sunshine.

When we spoke last she reminded me of the time when she, Jeff and I had played 45 holes of golf. This was on a par 3 course!

The mosquitoes were eating us alive when I begged them to play one more round. I don't know if they will ever be the same, the mosquitoes, the golf courses, the golf clubs or us. We were practically hysterical the last round, because suddenly everything was funny. As I recollect the scores were not that great but, boy did we have fun!

I regained almost all of my strength back walking those courses day after day. It was great mentally and physically for my body to get out there. I could not believe how weak a person becomes just lying around a hospital room for eight weeks at a time. We all know that I did more than lie around there though.

My doctor in Rochester happened to call one of the days to tell me my platelet count was low. The platelets are in the blood to help in clot formation. My counts were low enough that I needed a transfusion. When he finished the report, his final message was "I do hope you are not on the golf course." It was hilarious that he threw in the bit about golfing. He knew me too well! My red blood cell counts took a nosedive frequently; this meant that I needed numerous blood transfusions just to keep me going. So it shouldn't have been surprising that I was as weak as I was.

The only problem with this was the blood bank at the local hospital didn't have the supply that bigger cities had. That is part of the reason that leukemia patients were not treated there during that time. Couple that with the fact that the blood I needed had to be irradiated, this is where the blood needs to be exposed to a form of radiant energy (albeit heat, light or x-ray, for me it was through x-ray). The reason for that is x-rays in large amounts will destroy microorganisms of tissue cells that may have become cancerous. You never knew what types of cells the donor blood carried. Why allow any blood that may have suspicious cells be introduced to a person who is in remission from leukemia. Leukemia patients have already had cancer run rampant in their blood already; don't give them anymore.

That also was the reason why I could wait up to six hours for a transfusion; it needed to be sent from St. Paul, Minnesota. Keep in mind that in 1988 the Cancer Center in our hospital was still in

143

the embryonic stage. Since then a larger facility has been built that houses cancer patients for treatment. They provide the necessary treatments (chemotherapy, radiation therapy, transfusions, the list goes on and on). This was not yet available back then. So most of my care had to be done in Rochester. With the Cancer Center, I can now have any treatments done here at home and go to Rochester for checkups.

Golf had become important to me. I was frustrated that I couldn't even walk a mile without becoming winded when I first came home. The golf course every day became like my gymnasium. (Tiger Woods has nothing to be worried about though, so if you see him please tell him!) Most of the time on the shorter par 3 courses I would use a pull-cart. On the larger courses Jeff and I would break down and rent a cart, the kids used to enjoy going with us just to drive them.

I found out later that my daughter, Jennifer, hated the game of golf, being an athlete I was surprised to find that out. I guess I thought that if you were an athlete then you'd want to do it all. When we got the kids their own starter sets, we discovered that both Jennifer and Justin had one hell of a drive. They had all of this power in their arms from swimming year round. It was the short game that frustrated Jennifer. She would get on the green every time, but it took about eight strokes to putt. One day when she threw her clubs her father told her she was done. He meant only for that day, but she took it literally and totally quit. Justin, on the other hand, is perhaps now a better golfer than his father and I.

Once I returned to work, I used to take him and his friend to the course almost every day at about 2:30 p.m., on my way to work. Jeff would swing by to pick them up when he got off work at 4:30 p.m. At that time he would either pick them up or play a round with them.

He has continued interest in the game even today. He moved to Wisconsin with the company he has worked for since high school. While he was trying to decide whether or not to go, a component in the equation was that there was a four star golf course nearby. Interesting!

Chapter Twenty

NO ONE COULD EVER UNDERSTAND THE emotional roller coaster I was on during this time. Would I live or die? It depended on who you asked, some would tell you that I would make it, others may say that I bought the big one! There were those that couldn't deal with the fact I had cancer. A few of my friends got lost during that time, never finding their way back. They avoided me as if I had the plague.

This frustrated me; I wasn't any different because I had cancer. The only reason I could think of was that they didn't like bald headed women. In fact, I called one of my friends one day and asked her the question: "Don't you like me because I am bald? I haven't heard from you for a while." She stuttered and stammered for a moment, then told me that she had been busy. This was probably our last conversation. I decided that I wasn't going to chase anybody who didn't want to face me.

Realistically, people who are faced with cancer albeit a friend or family member that forces them to come to grips with their own mortality and that can be very scary. Along with the notion in his or her heads I wasn't going to survive, why would you hang around someone that is condemned to death? If they had hung on long enough they would have seen that I was a survivor. On the other hand, there were some new friends who came along. I had known them in passing at work. They have stuck out with me and are very close friends even today.

Death is hard for some to accept, including myself. I liked living too much! I felt that I'd grown from the experience while my old friends did not; they stood still. We no longer had the same things in common. I faced death, came to the edge so to speak, and they didn't.

I find that you need all kinds of support systems to fight cancer. I heard someone say once, that if they were ever again diagnosed with cancer they were sending postcards to everyone they knew. In order to circle the wagons, getting all their ducks in row or mustering the troops together, whichever phrase you choose you get the idea.

After my experience I know how important contact with people who care about you is. Even with all of its flaws there can be a Heaven on earth. It is all of what we make it. We can get up each morning thinking that life is a chore. Or we can become a Pollyanna and choose to find only the things that make us glad. Try playing the glad game sometime and you will be surprised how many things you have to make yourself glad.

It's like counting your blessings, and even when we are in the pit of depression there still are many blessings to be found. They are sometimes so close that we cannot see them though. I know for me that they were all right in my own back yard. I didn't have to go very far to search for the perfect place to be. It was here in my house, the one with a ceiling tile that is falling down in our family room, an unfinished bathroom, or a fireplace that doesn't work. But it is my home and I love it.

Another thing about my being home was that I once again found my husband to be my best friend. I know that some people would snicker at that, but it is true. I always told people that and even though we don't always agree we have a good relationship. We tell each other everything. We found early on that it was just

146

the two of us against the world, and if we stuck together it would all work out. Oh, believe me we have our little disagreements, we both are stubborn people, but they don't last long. We have been through quite a bit in our years of marriage, and a little squabble won't ever erase all we have shared.

One day as we drove up in front of our sitter's house, Jeff told me that she and her husband, along with several other people were setting up a benefit for me. This was to help defray the cost of my medical bills that were mounting higher each day.

They contacted many businesses, which donated items for prizes in a raffle. The local furniture store even donated a $900 sofa. It was too unbelievable! I didn't know half of these people, how would I ever repay them? Why did they do these things? I couldn't imagine what drove them to do this for me. I wasn't anyone special! But I was they said. You never realized how many people whose lives you touch until something like this happens. It kind of gives you a warm fuzzy feeling, doesn't it?

The benefit was held a week later on a Saturday and went off without a hitch. I was glad to still be at home to watch how it all came together. I walked around the gymnasium of the elementary school that held the benefit. Even though it was dreary outdoors, with a gentle spring rain, inside the warmth and love among these people made it seem like the sun was shining indoors. The weekend after the benefit I returned to Rochester for my next round of chemotherapy.

This is the Heartland, I thought! It's not just the crops we grow here, it's also the caring and gentle people we grow too. Coming together when someone is in need, finding they could make a difference in someone's life. The someone this time was me! It was truly a humbling experience. Thinking back on it now it still can bring me to tears. I thank God for bringing them into my life.

The week before the benefit I gave an interview to the local television station. They wanted to come and talk to me about what I had been through; it was also a way to advertise the benefit. It was different seeing myself on the television. As I watched the report on TV, I decided that a career on the big screen was not meant for me. I looked like the Goodyear blimp dressed in pink pants and a wild print shirt. On the top of my head rested a pink scarf of my own creation. To me I looked atrocious, but to the rest of the world I looked great. No one could believe that I had made it this far and for me all I was concerned about was how I looked to everyone. Isn't that a little too vain? I wasn't appearing in a Doris Day movie, where whenever you awoke you had perfect hair and makeup.

I knew that I wasn't a fashion model either. I knew that my skin had turned from an ivory tone to pure white. But when you don't have the red blood cells you need there is a tendency to pale up a bit. I am Italian, a small part anyway, and I had the most beautiful ivory colored skin. I didn't get any of the dark olive tones of the southern Italians near Sicily.

I always dreamed of being some raving Italian beauty with olive skin, dark brown eyes, and black hair. When I was in the Navy I had a friend who had just those traits I mentioned. Boy was I jealous of her! Not me I am pale, green-eyed, with dishwater blonde hair that I choose to highlight. Since chemotherapy my hair has gotten darker, as well as curlier. That is when I am not bald. Because of the tight curl I have I can't fathom the idea that people go out and get perms, I wish they had straightening salons. There I go again being vain.

I can remember telling the interviewer that I wanted to be around to raise my children and see my grandchildren grow up too. That was the truth all right, I wanted desperately to see the children grow into the fine adults I knew they would be. Naturally, I would like to see them have their own children, my grandchildren, some day. But that was far off in the future. You always want for your children, the things that you didn't have, to have the finer things in life. I only wanted for my children to feel love. Love in the surroundings that would teach them all that they needed to be able to survive in the world out there.

The phone didn't stop ringing after the interview I gave aired on the 6 o'clock news. The interview, the benefit and the people, it was all so great. It was then that I found out the people I worked with at the hospital held a bake sale. This too was to aid in meeting some of the financial burdens facing us.

I had insurance from my job; Jeff had me covered under his insurance policy too. All of this helped, yet you still manage to acquire a lot of bills even with insurance. That coupled with the fact that the disability I received was only 66 percent of my base pay. Then after paying out of pocket monthly insurance premiums it didn't leave much left over. After three months I had to pay the insurance premiums myself in order to carry my insurance. Jeff and I had managed to save some but it all was used to get us caught up on bills.

You never know how much you miss when your finances are cut in half, or how much you took for granted. We weren't wealthy by any means, but we were comfortable. We were able to pretty much buy what we wanted, still paying bills and have savings. Now we had to use savings to make ends meet.

The money we received from the hospital bake sale we put into CDs, which were set up for three months. The interest was around 9% at the time and gave me enough return on my investment that it made it worthwhile. The reason why three months is that I never knew what would happen, and at the time three months seemed like a safe increment of time for me to plan into the future. I was afraid to not plan for the future, as well as I was afraid to plan for the future. I realize that it doesn't make much sense, but not much about what was happening to me made sense.

I didn't understand why I had to worry about what went on in the months ahead, just that it was important for me to make future plans. Not just any kind of plans, just something to look forward to! I guess I thought that if I had something to do months in advance I would go on living. I know that this sounds a little weird, but I find myself planning ahead even now.

I kind of ran around in circles in a panic searching desperately for something to hang on to. I would make these plans like, in three months we will go to Minneapolis. Or maybe in one year we

149

will take a long trip, I was afraid that this was maybe too much of a stretch. I felt that if I planned for things in the future it meant I wasn't sitting waiting for the other shoe to drop. If I didn't make plans then I was sitting in limbo nervously waiting, I just couldn't have that. I needed to be busy doing things. It was as though I was driven by this demon I had inside of me, the damn cancer demon. Pushing me forward, onward no matter what I would do just to keep busy.

Chapter Twenty-one

WHEN I WENT TO ROCHESTER FOR the next round of chemotherapy, things were pretty much the same as it had been a few short weeks before. The nausea, pain, vomiting, diarrhea, blood transfusions, fevers, weakness, and let us not forget the bone marrow biopsies.

When they felt I met all of their criteria they cut me loose. This time I had two weeks cut off of my stay, making it only six weeks of captivity. Once again golf became my gym, simply picking up where I had left off, one could say golf was a safe haven for me. I believed if I could play golf then I wasn't sick. Can you see that the mind was playing a big part in my sense of well-being? If I could walk a golf course then I must be okay, right? This is the part where you just say yes, and agree with me!

After that round came a third and final round of treatment. I shouldn't need to spell it all out for you, should I? Before I went home that time I was able to get my Hickman out. Hooray! Yet I did have to go back about six weeks later to have a bone marrow harvest. What is a harvest you ask? That is when they gather enough marrow to store, for you in case I would ever need a transplant.

151

If they felt I would need a transplant sometime in the future, they needed to harvest my bone marrow while I was in remission. I didn't have a related donor. My brother and I were half brother and sister with different fathers. This meant I would receive what is called an autologous transplant; this meant my own marrow would be given back to me. I would then be counted as one of the first autologous transplants at the Mayo Clinic.

Once they have the marrow, they add DMSO to it, which is an abbreviation for dimethyl sulfoxide, which is used as a preservative. They draw the marrow with several syringes from each hip (iliac crest). Thank God for general anesthesia! There was no way I would sit still for that while I was awake. Not that there would ever be a transplant, you see I insisted that I would never need it. Once I was healed from the harvest I was able to finally go back to work. It was one of the few hurdles I felt I had left to conquer.

It was June when we went back for my bone marrow harvest. We met with my doctor at the clinic before I was admitted to the hospital. We had the project he ordered me to complete with us; it had been matted and framed. I gave it to him as a gift for saving my life. He took it to the BMT unit where it hung there for a few years before finding its way to his office wall. I believed I surprised him with it, but you could see how happy he was with it.

I discovered that just as there were stages of an illness that patients go through, I believe there are also stages of survival. These are a few more stages to be tacked on besides the ones that deal with learning how to survive. Feeling no guilt for surviving when others did not live and learning how to be free to live again. There were two people who I had come to know while I was going through treatment that weren't as lucky as I was. They didn't survive their leukemia. Because they had such full lives ahead of them I was at times ashamed that I lived and they didn't.

Ridding myself of all these little fears I had built up along the way. I know you wonder what all these have to do with surviving, but believe me anyone that is battling a life-threatening illness like cancer knows what I am talking about.

Little by little I gained back the control that I felt I had lost over my life. The time that I was robbed of would never return. There was no turning the page back to where the whole mess began. There have been written many articles and books that dealt with the different stages of the death and dying. For those of us that do survive, there should be another book titled *Life and Living*. In death and dying I have seen some people get themselves stuck in one stage or another, or sometimes the stages aren't followed in exact order. You see when I was first told that I had cancer; I immediately went into the first stage, the one of disbelief. I couldn't believe that such a thing could happen to anyone, let alone me. I kept thinking it was all a mistake.

I became a nurse to take care of other people that were sick and dying, it wasn't supposed to be me! I wasn't supposed to get cancer. I was supposed to be there for the really sick people. For some unknown reason I got handed the wrong script, right? Is this life or a play, whichever it may be I request to have this act deleted! Okay?

Sometimes people are given someone else's diagnosis, I just knew that this was to be in my case. All the people that I had ever taken care of that had cancer were really sick. I didn't feel sick (other than the recurring sore throat) so I was positive that I couldn't have cancer. The sad thing is that every stage I went through no one ever said that a mistake had been made in my case. They only continued telling me I had cancer, no one was sure what kind just that I had it.

The next stage that I went through was anger. Well let me tell you…I have had anger burning inside of me from the beginning and at times still have anger now. When I was growing up I was always told that anger wasn't a good thing. In fact, I tell my son that he must get his anger under control all the time. I had a hard time believing that it was and is okay for me to be angry. On the other hand though I also believe that some of that anger is the reason why I am here today to tell my story. Remember I was spunky. So you could say, I got damn mad! The anger I was experiencing was the kind that drove me to survive. That along with the sense of humor that I have could be what saved me. I was angry enough to decide from the start that I would live. I would not accept this plight without a fight.

There had been enormous changes in my life. I had always been afraid to say what was on my mind before, a kind of *Casper Milk Toast*. Or, I would have asked my mother to move out that first December when Jeff gave me his ultimatum. Or, told Jeff that I don't like ultimatums for that matter. Always speaking what is on my mind. To my family I have never been honest with my feelings, so I allowed myself to get into situations that hurt me. I am who I am! Since cancer I gave myself the freedom to be me! To live my life the way I wanted to, only remembering to live it to the fullest.

The next stage was bargaining; I didn't entertain that one for too long. You see I had heard of people that bargained with God. Asking for more time, when the time they had asked for came about they willingly laid down their lives and died. If I bargained for anything it would be for another one hundred years. Why put limits on anything in life, right? Why put limits on God?

I have been told of many people just wanting to see their children raised, or their grandchildren married or until we get a better President. When they get to those milestones they are willing to go peacefully. Not me, I wouldn't spend much time in the bargaining stage, I will ask for forever. Each day is a wonderful surprise, just waiting to unlock the door to its treasures. Each one of us is given twenty-four hours in a day and it is up to us to use it.

Sense of loss and depression make up the next stage. Well I am not sure where I am as far as this stage is concerned. I was depressed at times, why? Mostly, because I couldn't handle the isolation I had been feeling. I was sitting idle and the entire world was passing me by. I didn't want to miss as much of what was going on as I did.

My family simply continued with their lives while I wasn't there. I was jealous because they had lives. I wasn't sure what it was I had, I just knew I was depressed over the loss I was experiencing. I couldn't work; I couldn't do much of anything, just sit in my room on the BMT unit and watch the world fly by. Sitting here and writing this now even makes me a little depressed just thinking about what has all happened since that first day. The sense of loss is the time I missed from it all, from my job, my life, my family and the world in general.

The final stage is acceptance; well in a sense I guess you could say I experienced some of this. I finally accepted that I had cancer, but that is about all I ever accepted. I would not allow myself the acceptance of the fact I was going to die. I was going to live!

It's just how you see things. For me I don't say that I am dying from leukemia, I say that I am living with leukemia. How do you view a glass of water that is not up to the top? Do you see it as half empty or half full? I choose to see it half full, that is living on the positive side. There is too much in the world that is negative I don't go looking for it in my own back yard. I will never accept the enemy; I will not go through this stage, because I don't accept anything other than the fact once I had cancer.

I mentioned that I not only went through those stages, but that I had a few more that I had to learn to go through on my road to survival. One of these was feeling free to live again. I guess that must sound strange after my last few sentences on how I didn't accept death. I had so many people think that I wasn't going to make it that I had to be the one to stay positively focused. I can't tell you how afraid I was to go and live again. I didn't know that I had merely existed up until now. I was just going through the motions never taking it all in.

Most people go through the routine of their day forgetting to take a close look at what they truly have. No one realizes how swiftly things can end; life can be taken from you. I cannot drive home the point enough the fact is we are only mortal. We live our lives in this day and age on rigid schedules. We all have to be in different places at different times. Does anyone have family meals at any time during the day? I ask the question is any of it really important? Or better yet, ask what is important? Don't lose yourselves in the rat race and lose who you are.

I could have gone back to work sooner, but my doctor restricted my lifting after the bone marrow harvest to no more than ten pounds, the restriction was for ten days. Our employee health nurse said that I must wait the full ten days before I could return to work. She wouldn't let me come back under any circumstances, even though my head nurse promised that she would make sure that I wouldn't do any heavy lifting for those ten days, the answer was still no. What a jerk! No I shouldn't say that, she is only protecting the hospital as well as me. And I guess rules are rules, besides I had no real choice in the matter.

The only thing is that I laugh now because I see people come back to work all the time with a lifting restriction and they don't even bat an eyelash. Oh well, another ten days wouldn't be all that bad after all I had already waited six months. I have already told you that patience is not a virtue of mine, and I seem to be tested all the time by this.

I can remember the day I returned to work as if it were yesterday. It was hot and sultry outside, anyone living in Iowa can tell you that the air kind of hangs around you. If you have never experienced August in the Midwest you don't know what you're missing. It is so hot you can barely breathe, it is like living in a greenhouse all of the time. But that is why we are known for the land of tall corn. Everything grows here, and I am sure that if you ask the farmers you will be told especially the weeds. I am battling the weeds now in my raspberry patch.

I was scared to death about returning. I made one of my friends come to my house and ride in to work with me. I realize that this might sound a bit childish but I had myself convinced I couldn't face these people alone. When we rode up in the elevator together I had butterflies in my stomach the size of robins doing flip-flops and loopy-loops. As we entered the unit I felt like I could just faint, my hands were all clammy and cold. If you ask my husband though he will tell you my hands are always cold so this wasn't anything really new for me.

As soon as I saw everyone and they saw me, we hugged and cried. Believe me that was all I needed to feel more relaxed. How could I ever have been afraid to return to these people? How foolish I was. These people had become like family to me, we had gone through this ordeal together. They were super. I never realized until that moment how important we all are to one another. We are not islands, we are not alone in life, and we need each other in spite of ourselves. These people gave me something to come back to.

I was finally out of the scarves; my hair was all of a half an inch long. And dark let me tell you; it was much darker than I had ever remembered my own hair to be. At least what I thought my true hair color was. I had bleached it with highlighting for so many years, who knew what my natural color really was? Believe me not even my hairdresser was sure.

It was quite funny the day I returned and one of the RNs came to me and said, "Weren't you surprised when your hair came in so dark? It's really too bad, your hair was so blonde." I just answered her "NO," walked away and laughed to myself. She actually thought I was a true blonde, either it was the best dye job ever or she was a little on the flaky side not to realize that I was a bottle blonde not a natural one.

Speaking of my hairdresser let me tell you that I was embarrassed to see him. Why? Because this man out of the goodness of his heart had purchased a wig for me, similar in color to what my own hair was. Remember that when he came to Rochester to cut off the golden tresses he took some home with him to have a wig made.

My golfing buddy and I stopped to see him after he had my wig come in. It was too hard for me to see this wig cut in the same style like the hair I had lost, let alone to wear it like that. I wouldn't let him see me bald, when I had the wig in my hand I made him go around the corner until I got it on my head. He cut it in a bob length to my shoulders, and at first I liked it. It was great walking around the mall with hair again. I found that fewer people stared. When he was all done we left.

We then went to a matinee at the mall theater; Patrick Swayze was starring in *Roadhouse*. I'd watch Patrick Swayze in anything, but that's an entirely different story. About halfway through the movie my head started itching. I was getting crazy trying not to knock the hair off my head while I was scratching. Every time I reached up and scratched, the wig would rock back and forth like a seesaw. It was about falling off from all the commotion. If I had only had a scarf with me I would have taken off the wig and put that on instead. When the movie was over, I found my wig had shifted enough that my bangs were practically in my right ear. I am glad I made that discovery before leaving the darkness of the movie theatre.

When I got home that afternoon I could hardly wait to finally remove it, and sad to say I never wore it again. That is why I was embarrassed to see my hairdresser. I didn't want to appear ungrateful for all he had done for me. He is a wonderful person and I will always be indebted to him for everything he did, but I am not a wig person. Perhaps it comes from all the years watching my mother wear them when I was a child. She had quite the assortment of the silly things too. I hated them then and having to wear one because I was bald I hated them even more.

Being back at work was as if I hadn't been gone for six months; I often refer to that time as my sabbatical. I was able to jump right back into the routine of the floor with very little problem. The only thing that I was having a little difficult time with was IV starts, it had been six months since I started an IV and I was quite nervous my first time out. I was nervous for both the patient and me. The first time I was able to start an IV successfully I wanted to jump for joy. I was good at starting them before, I don't mean to brag but even while I was in the Navy I was able to start them with little problem. I was happy to see that nothing had changed much during my absence, that the six months barely made a difference.

Everyone including the doctors I knew told me how good I looked. I don't know how they could say that with a straight face, by this time I had already started my upward swing of weight gain. I had lost weight when I was in the hospital from my many rounds of chemotherapy. But after that I gave myself the license to eat whatever I wanted as well as all that I wanted. I ate all the time. I was afraid of turning into the image I always had of the typical cancer patient.

When it was all totaled I was approximately one hundred and twenty-five pounds over my initial weight. At least that is how much overweight I was the day I walked into Weight Watchers. Sad but true, it was like I was carrying around another person on my back. That is more than what my daughter weighs, so it was just like carrying her around with me all the time. I shouldn't be surprised that I was not able to climb even my basement stairs without being winded.

I don't remember when I started to put on weight while growing up. I just remember always needing to watch my weight. I watched all right, as it climbed into the stratosphere. My mother who has always been slender used to promise me a new wardrobe if I could take off the weight. It was as if it fell on deaf ears.

They say just like quitting smoking, that you will lose weight when you are ready. This upward trend went on until I finally was disgusted enough to start Weight Watchers. That is all finally behind me. I have belonged to Weight Watchers for a year and have managed to lose at this point fifty-eight pounds. I realize that it will take me awhile longer to get the rest of it off but with continued effort and belief in myself I know that I will attain my goal weight.

My only problem is like I told you before that I have this lack of patience. So that tells you I have little patience with the weight loss thing too. I get really irritated and I find myself eating because I am mad. Or if I have a good weight loss one week, the next week I use that as an excuse to eat. I thought that if I had been good, that I then could splurge. It is something that I battle daily and even though I have my good and bad days I am confident someday I will make it to my goal weight.

Chapter Twenty-two

MY HEAD NURSE CALLED ME INTO her office one day and asked me to take the charge nurse job on the evening shift. I couldn't believe that she had that much faith in my abilities to think I would be able to do a good enough job. I was truly amazed that I was chosen. So let me go over this in my mind, I was gone for six months, back to work only about one month and asked to take charge. Somehow it confuses me even now.

Once I said yes, I spent the next three days learning what I needed to know from the other charge nurse. She had taken a job in the ICU/CCU unit. It was great for me, but I hated to see her go. I knew she would do well in the units, because she was a good nurse. The other charge nurse was staying on as a staff nurse.

I took on my new role with an attitude of fear. I was afraid of making a sudden move in the wrong direction for fear of being reported. The shoes that those two left behind were going to be hard to fill. I was afraid I couldn't fit the bill, as my predecessors had. Oh-oh! It was stress revisited! I believed it would be hard to establish my own rapport. I knew that everyone would be watching me and waiting for me to make a mistake and eventually fail. I myself was waiting for me to fail, I guess I was so insecure in my role that I just knew I wouldn't do a good job.

Wrong move, you never wait in anticipation to fail at anything, your job, marriage, parenting, or life in general. You never just sit and wait to see if it all works out. Just as I tell my children, if you can look back on something and say that you have given your best then how can you fail at anything you do? That is what I preach anyway, just ask the kids. Remember, it's do as I say—not do as I do!

Things from here seemed to go along well over the next few months, the staff in their places and me dealing with the mounting paranoia that went along with my placement into the charge nurse position. I don't think that I would have been half as paranoid if I had gotten the position because the other charge people were moved. You do realize that the only one that was uncomfortable was myself. No one else seemed to be as bothered by this as I was.

In time the stress of the new position I was in, coupled with the tension of my fears of leukemia coming back, the inevitable did take place. It was around Thanksgiving that I noticed the first bump. On my chest again, they began to appear one by one that alone should have been the tip-off, because that is the place the rash showed up the first time. I guess deep in my soul I knew that my leukemia was alive again, like a sleeping dragon awakening, just waiting to devour me. In my head I kept on rationalizing it all away. They weren't there! I wasn't going to have to go back into the hospital and go through it all over again! I cannot tell you the fear that gripped me most of the time during these few days trying desperately to hold on, even now after all these years I still panic when I see a rash...anywhere on my body.

I didn't tell Jeff that the bumps had returned for nearly a week, not until there were two of them anyway. He didn't want to believe that we could be heading for another disaster. He continued to deny it all for about another week himself.

Finally, he came to his senses, thank God...one of us had to! He called my doctor in Rochester. You see I myself would never

161

have called him. By now it was the middle of December, and because of our delay I could have lost my life. Why not call you ask? Because I was not going to go through that hell I went through again willingly. I'm not a complete fool! I was terrified! I hope that doesn't surprise you. Naturally, the good doctor told him that he wanted to see me the following week, on a Wednesday. I guess for a while I thought if he didn't want to see me for another week it couldn't be that bad, right?

It was a shame because when I saw him last it had been in October. He told me that he would let me go three months before I needed to see him again. I was going to be able to go through the holidays, having a good time because he told me it would be okay. I wasn't supposed to have this happen. How had I failed? What did I do wrong? I knew that it must have been because of something I had done. I was headed for the biggest fall of all now and didn't even know it.

That noon hour when Jeff came home for lunch he told me what he had done. Jeff has had to tell me many things in our lives together but I honestly think that this was the hardest yet. "I called the doctor this morning."

With that sentence I freaked totally out. I came unglued! I started yelling at him. "How could you? Why did you do that? They aren't the same kind of bumps! This is not the same rash! I just know that it isn't the same thing," I screamed at him, while I cried uncontrollably. Then suddenly I calmed down. "I will go to the stupid appointment and I will be fine. You'll see." I talked as though I had control over the whole thing, when in essence I didn't have much control over anything since this mess began. I would show them all, and then I could tell them "I told you so!"

After Jeff left I got into my car. I drove all around town for about twenty minutes while I sobbed. I found myself in East Park; this is a nearby park, only about five blocks from my front door. It is one of the most beautiful parks I have ever seen. I just sat there; I looked at the trees and the sky. It was a cold December afternoon, it hadn't snowed yet, but it was a blustery day nonetheless. Through the gray sky I saw a hint of sun shining through. I felt that it was a sign from God that I would be okay. I didn't know at the time I was right, I would be okay. Again I needed to muster up the strength I needed to fight one more battle…the one for my life, once again!

The days waiting for my appointment were days that made me feel numb again. It was almost like a reenactment of what had transpired earlier that year. I had my work to run to and hide from. I had my family to comfort me. I had my children who needed me to care for them. I loved them all so dearly, the thought of them having to suffer anymore made me sad. It was so hard to tell them that day that I would have to go back to Rochester sooner than I had planned.

They weren't dumb. They knew that after my visit in October the doctor had told me I didn't need to return to see him until after the holidays, sometime in January. Well, this was only December so they knew that something was not right. I hated to tell them. I just sat there at the table making light of the whole thing while Jeff explained that I needed to go back to have a rash checked on. I reassured them that this was not the same rash that I had earlier; Jeff simply sat there saying not a word while I spun my web of lies.

He was as convinced as I was that I was going to have to have more chemotherapy and maybe I would not come back, for a long while once again. You see my husband has always been the level-headed one. He lived in the real world; I often chose to live in the clouds. Sometimes I could take him to new heights and other times he would pull me down to walk with him. I tell our friends that he has always been my perfect balance on life's path. So when I discounted the thought that I would never be faced with this again he kept trying to prepare me for this very thing.

Still the look of horror that appeared on their little faces made me die inside, I don't really think I fooled them either. I had a hard time choking back my tears, but managed to tell them when I returned that evening we would go out for pizza. They lightened up a little bit because you didn't know that my children are champion pizza eaters, did you?

163

You see that the way to the heart of my children is through their stomachs. You might laugh at that but I swear my daughter has a pit someplace that she deposits it all into. She can put most adult males to shame, with her enormous appetite. I would be concerned if she didn't have the amount of activity in her life that she does. She is a swimmer and is on the swim team in our town, so she spends many hours in the pool. And so I am not as afraid of her ferocious appetite. What amazes me even more is that when she isn't swimming she isn't hungry.

I'll never forget the day she came home from a classmate's birthday party, they had a barbecue in their back yard. She was just as pleased as she could be that she had eaten five hamburgers. "More than anyone else." I tried to explain to her that the idea was for her to celebrate a birthday not to eat them out of house and home. I'm sure they were happy to see her go home before they would have to purchase a side of beef to feed her. She isn't one for sweets and junk food though, that's my son, and so it is all nutritional food, just in major quantities.

On the other hand my son is the junk food king. He hates most items that are good for you, but you give him cake or pizza and you'll have yourself a friend for life. Justin also loves breakfast and a half a box of Lucky Charms is usually a normal size breakfast for him, now as a young adult he uses a bowl I use to make the family salads in. Jennifer dislikes breakfast, at least the traditional breakfast that I was raised on, that she was raised on for that matter. Yogurt, cheese, and cold pizza make up her early morning meals. It is hard to believe that they are as opposite as they are. They are so different that it is fun to watch them grow, I want to stay around to see how it all comes out.

It was Wednesday, December 13, 1989, when we drove up to the clinic in the dark of the morning like all the other times. I remember telling the children that I would see them that evening and we would have more pizza. I knew that I wouldn't be coming home that evening, I looked at the house with a look like I wanted to take it all in. I wanted to memorize every inch of this place I called home because I didn't know if and when I would be returning.

The drive was in silence, the same type of silence that we felt the first time we took this trip. I kept trying to sleep; I knew that sleep could be my escape. I didn't have to think or deal with any of this and I wouldn't have to if I could just go to sleep. Oh, God, no! I am so scared! Help me now please! That is all I kept repeating to myself over and over.

I sat there so close to Jeff I wanted desperately for him to take me in his arms and love me. Hold me and make this all go away. Have I told you lately that I love you, Jeff? Have I told you enough times that I could never have gone through this all without you? Have we made love enough times that I will never forget every inch of your body and the gentleness of your touch?

Isn't it sad that it's not until we hit the really rough times that we appreciate the things we have. That I had to come to this point in my life to really see what kind of a man I had fallen in love with. I had to almost die before I appreciated what I would lose. Why, God, do we not learn these lessons the easy way? Why do we have to nearly die to finally appreciate life? That you have to almost lose your life in order to learn how to live?

Jeff will never know how hard it was to not just stop that day; if he wouldn't have been with me I don't think I could have done it on my own. You see I must again admit that I am a coward. I hate pain, especially my own. Now having experienced what I did the first time didn't make me any braver. It just made me an informed coward.

We arrived at our destination in the early part of the morning. The sun was barely up as we came over the hill with the Mayo Clinic buildings off in the distance. So big, even from eight miles away. I could see the gray concrete and the steel, it was so cold and impersonal. Suddenly I thought to myself, *I wonder if the lady with half glasses is signing people in for their lab tests.* I wanted desperately to give her a hard time, but I was too depressed and too afraid to even play any games with her that day.

I just wanted to get this over with, I wanted to go to the doctor's office and have him tell Jeff and I to stop panicking. But he didn't. This time he had concern on his face as he examined me and looked at the bumps. He insisted that we go to have one of them biopsied. That is until he called for my lab work, he had tears in his eyes when they read him the results. I could see him swallow hard as he hung up the phone. I thought to myself, *Let's make it easy on the old boy, I will tell him my diagnosis this time.* "It's back, isn't it?" I asked. My voice calm yet the tears were streaming down my face. All he did was nod. I stared into his eyes, looking into the soul of this man and told him, "Just fix it!" With that he took my hand and nodded.

I didn't know until I was going to my unit, after the entire admission process that I had not been the only visitor to the clinic, not the only one to relapse. Sheila was back too. Who was Sheila? She was my doctor's other favorite patient. We both had the same kind of leukemia but she was treated with the other protocol, which was different from the one I had.

When Sheila came to the hospital, her marrow on admission was packed with blasts (immature cells). She was young, probably denying like I did that her leukemia had returned. I would've or could've been in the same boat had I not had Jeff watching over me, and on his own called the doctor. Sheila had been away at school, doing whatever nineteen-year-olds do.

She came back after waiting a lot longer than I had before she admitted her leukemia had returned. During the time Sheila was alive, she had learned how to live life to the fullest. Though she would not survive this time, she had lived. It is something a lot of us cannot say we have done; even making it to the age of one hundred, some of us only exist.

I was in denial to the nth degree; I didn't want to believe that this had started all over. The walk through the tunnels into the hospital was like walking down the last mile. I was feeling like such a failure that I was sure I was going in but, I was not so sure that I would be coming out. I was really scared now.

Jeff and I were silent, we were afraid to look at each other for fear that we would both fall apart. How were we going to tell the children? How was Jeff going to tell the children? My God I made promises to them for pizza, I've let them down again. As the elevator door opened and the people congregated to get on for the next ride to the top, I saw a familiar face in the crowd. It was one of the nurses from the BMT unit. At first when our eyes met he had the look of I know you. Then when it dawned on him who I was he was shocked. You could tell he knew why I was there, he asked anyway. "Jeanine, what are you doing here? Coming for a visit?" He tried to joke with me. I just turned my head to the wall and sobbed.

"It's back, make it better."

Chapter Twenty-three

THE ELEVATOR STOPPED ON THE EIGHTH floor. As I looked around I had a feeling in the pit of my stomach like I always got when I was on a Ferris wheel. This place was too familiar, the elevators, the halls and the highly polished linoleum floors beneath my feet. My heart started pounding faster as if it would jump out of my chest, my hands were getting cold and clammy, and I thought I could faint. I was dazed like a deer caught in headlights. It reminded of the day I was told I had some form of cancer, which was the beginning of this whole nightmare. I guess that I got there on autopilot, because some of the things are sketchy.

The escort led us down the hall to the BMT unit; I noticed the nurses that I knew (and liked) were all on duty that day. Slowly, Jeff and I walked around the nurse's station heading to my room.

The nurses tried to joke with me, but I didn't find anything amusing at the time. This whole thing made me sad and disappointed. That is all I could think about. Where did I go wrong? What hadn't I done right? And then there is the classic, why me? To that, my friend, I now answer, why not me? It is a little hard to write those words because it is so contradictory to what we all think. Why would anyone be thankful that they have cancer? Being older and hopefully wiser, the most unfortunate part is that I had to learn my lessons over several years. Sometimes I guess I learn better when I hit my head against a brick wall a few times. Don't we all?

Once we were in my room, the staff left me alone for a while. I could process all the incoming messages my mind was receiving as I started to settle in. I was reeling with the news of my relapse. When the shock started to wear off, all I could do was cry. Jeff and I didn't say much of anything to each other. I often think now that he would've loved at this point to tell me, *I told you so!* He must be thinking I put all my eggs in one basket with all the big talk I did about my leukemia not ever coming back, or saying I would not ever need a transplant. All this changed when I spotted the stupid rash on my chest, signaling it had returned. I failed, didn't I? My main focus at this moment was the feeling of failure.

When the nurses finally came back in to my room, it was time to do the paperwork that needed to be done on admission. The resident and Chief Resident then followed them; they were there to examine me. These residents were new to me and they told me I had become a kind of legend on the unit, so they said they were happy to finally meet me. They said that the staff talked about me all the time. If I would not have been in such a down mood I may have thought being infamous could be fun. Not now, not at this time. I was too scared.

Finally the bone marrow nurses tracked me down; they are like hound dogs—relentlessly seeking out their prey. Of course I was to have one of those awful things, they wanted to see how involved my marrow was. I could rationalize this out with little difficulty, especially being a nurse, but getting it past my brain and to my heart was a more difficult maneuver. I really believe I should have had them start carving my initials in my backside from the start. I would have had one hell of a design back there by now.

169

I was given some pre-medication so at least the pain would be somewhat tolerable. Once they were finished I drifted off to sleep. Jeff sat quietly next to my bed watching TV. I'm sure he wasn't even seeing what was on the tube in front of him; he just continued channel-surfing. I think in his mind he was back home, having to tell the children one more time that I was sick. I believe that he had a much harder task than I. He had to deal with their questions and those sweet little faces. I simply would be sent to la-la land via the Ativan express.

When I woke I started mulling everything over in my mind, it was going to start all over the nausea, vomiting, diarrhea, chemotherapy, a new Hickman, all of it. This time I was going to receive high doses of Ara-C as my chemotherapy regimen. I would get the chemo twice a day for five days. All I could remember of the drug was that this was the stuff that made my joints ache, that was with a lower dose. I couldn't imagine what getting high doses would do.

I never saw my doctor again until he returned from his vacation (not really, I heard his mother was ill). He needed to go and think what his next move was going to be. His two prize patients had relapsed, he wasn't clear what he should do, transplant or no transplant. Quite the dilemma I guess! I didn't think it needed much thought; I just wanted it fixed whatever it took. I wanted my life back! I couldn't continue this lollygagging around, I had to dust myself off and get back on the merry-go-round called life.

Believe it or not I wanted desperately to get back to work. It's funny how we all complain about our jobs, including myself, but when it is taken away from me, and not by choice mind you, it was all I could think about. Going back and caring for people that were really sick. In my mind I wasn't as sick as I really was. I had and still have a tendency to deny just how serious this all was. I was at a point where I did not want to be told my prognosis either. I wanted simply to live…Sometimes I think that if I would have been told the statistics regarding my condition, I might have become a statistic myself.

The same two residents came to my room the next day, with the results of my bone marrow biopsy. They said that eight-seven percent of my marrow had leukemia cells. It wasn't as bad as if I had come in with a blast crisis, but it was bad enough.

Later on the second day I went to surgery to have another Hickman placed. This time they put it on the opposite side. Which was okay, in fact I told the surgeons where would be the best position to not bother me when I wore a bra. You may think I could go braless, let me tell you that this is not an option for me. To say I am well endowed is an understatement; believe me I am not bragging I am complaining. I'm not as large as Dolly Parton but who knows we could share some of the same genes. I simply thought that if I told the doctors where the Hickman should go we could save a lot of frustration, especially on my part.

Soon after all this was done and over I started my chemotherapy. Oh, the nectar of the gods served to me straight from the pharmacy. It wasn't long after I started the treatment that my joints started to ache. Especially my ankles, walking became quite a challenge, I had to navigate the floor before I could take a step, I felt like I was wearing those big clown shoes and trying to walk in them. The nurses requested the doctor to start me on a morphine drip by IV the pain was so bad. Now not only was I in la-la land during the chemotherapy I was in la-la all day long.

Then the waiting game for my blood counts to drop and then to have them come back up again. When my counts were at the lowest, it was during that time I would get sick. During this treatment I not only had joint pain I also was experiencing numbness and tingling in my hands and feet. In fact, it was hard to hold a pen so my signature left a lot to be desired, glad I was only writing thank-you cards and not signing any official documents. Can you say illegible?

Keeping in mind this is December and we all know who comes that month. Yeah, Santa Claus! And come to town he did, my husband all dressed up in his Santa costume drove the ninety miles from home to surprise me. My family: Jennifer, Justin, Jeff, my mother, my brother and his fiancée all joined me on the BMT unit for a Christmas celebration.

It truly was the most wonderful time we shared together; in fact, if you were to ask any one of the participants they would tell you it was probably the best Christmas they had. We laughed, joked, ate, drank, opened presents, and were full of holiday cheer.

My mother had decorated my room well. I had tabletop Christmas trees, garland, ornament, lights and even some tinsel. My mother had called one of the local hotels that advertised complete holiday meals catered. We had the whole nine yards too, turkey, dressing, mashed potatoes, cranberries, corn, dessert and even yams with marshmallows. Being the New Ager he was, Jeff shot videos of the whole escapade with my mother's camcorder. We've watched the tape through the years; even to this day it still makes us laugh. The kids are naturally much older, so their focal point is just how young they were "back then."

The best medicine and Christmas present I could have gotten was being able to hold my babies again. They smelled and felt wonderful to me. Jeff and I never wanted the children to come to visit me whenever I was really sick. At their ages we thought it might frighten them too much. Instead we settled for telephone calls and visits only when I was doing well.

My brother teased his fiancée about her school colors were periwinkle and taupe. He also helped Justin organize his new baseball and football cards he had gotten as gifts. His fiancée was telling Jennifer about the high points of diamonds and gold. Jeff put his entire Santa garb back on and visited other patients that were well enough to have a visit from Santa. My mother was tidying thing up and keeping everything in nice order. I just sat back on my bed soaking it all in. Just before they left we all played some board games laughing until we cried.

If I knew then, what I know now, I would've signed us all up for family counseling when it was over. But I didn't, so we lived and learned the hard way, each in our own private hell. The children we thought were doing so well, it wasn't until later that

172

we discovered they had suppressed all of their feelings and fears. The things we repress will eventually surface or as they say, come back to haunt you. It can take on many forms: headaches, achy muscles, depression, or a general feeling of the blahs. Think about it and answer truthfully: have any of you ever experienced any of these symptoms? If so, then what might you be repressing? (Kind of a "What's in your wallet?" thing.)

We all laugh and make jokes about it now, but then not much was funny. Not anymore, in fact I was and am always accused of not being serious enough. The world continued to turn and life went on and I had to make a choice, to become an active participant or curl up and die. All through my life, giving up never seemed to be an option in anything I chose to do. So you can figure out what my decision was.

My room was a nice big one, so at least I didn't feel claustrophobic; in fact, I had an exercise cycle in my room. One of the nurses, who was at the top of my "hit parade," told me a story about a patient who was riding on the exercise cycle. His IV tubing got caught around the pedal and out came the Hickman. It was told to me as a warning, I didn't peddle around much after that, the last thing I wanted was to rip this awful thing out and they may have to put it back in.

It wasn't long before they started to remodel the BMT unit, so they moved everything including the patients to another unit during the renovation. The number of patients were two, remember it was Christmas so the census was low. I always remember when I was working over holidays the census would drop markedly.

It was nice because any staff who were scheduled to work the holidays could opt to put their name on a list for what was called a "low census day." The same was true here. The only drawback being if you truly counted on a low census day, going so far as to make plans, it could be denied.

Then your plans would be thwarted. This is not a negative attitude just a realistic one, I've seen it happen far too often. It went something like this; two or three days before the date you

173

want off the census would be low, so you put your name on a list to hopefully have that date off. Only to find your unit either had six or seven admissions or someone had their name in ahead of you. I never counted on low census days; I found it never paid off, especially over the holidays. Through all my stays in the hospital, the hardest times were holidays, followed by nights, and weekends. Everything was much too quiet for me, and the silence was deafening.

The rooms on this new unit we moved to, during the renovation, were definitely not meant for lengthy visits. My room would barely fit two chairs in it for company to sit down. I no longer had my exercise cycle, and I couldn't watch my geese come and go. To say the quarters were cramped was an understatement. I do believe that there is more room on board a ship or submarine where they sleep three bunks high. I learned what the meaning of being flexible or to coin a phrase, going with the flow was.

I was starting to feel better so I was also getting spunkier. I gave the doctors and nurses a run for their money. I was back to joking with them, we renamed all the residents in the dog and pony show. I had all I could do to contain my laughter.

New Year's always follows Christmas and so it was true this year. I remember one of the nurses I became friends with said he would bring in some sparkling grape juice, so we could toast in the New Year. He would be working the night shift and I definitely was a captive audience. I also believe I was the only patient under seventy at the time.

As you could have predicted, the unit got busy that night, it was after midnight when I finally came out of my room looking for my date. Had I been stood up? After I found him we shared a glass of the bubbly. There is something that has stuck in the back of mind that he said that night as we raised our glasses high. "I guarantee you that neither one of us will be here next New Year's Eve." It hit me like a bolt of lightning, I didn't know what he meant by that statement and I was too afraid to ask. He must have seen the panic in my eyes because he clarified himself quickly by adding, "I won't be working and you will be at home." Phew was what I thought next, I could breathe again. That made me a little nervous and even though he did clarify himself I still to this day remember those words.

After we grabbed our quick drink and gave a quick toast I walked back to my room slowly, my hands stuffed deeply in my bathrobe pockets. When I looked back to again say good night and happy New Year he was already scurrying into another patient's room. Here it was New Year's Eve and I was again alone. I missed my family more at that time than I had up to then. A new year meant new beginnings and we were apart. They were planning on coming up the next day, which was some consolation, but it wasn't the same. As I laid my head on my pillow that night I closed my eyes and tried to remember the faces of my family as I started to cry. It was nearly two in the morning before I finally fell asleep.

Jeff and the kids along with my mother arrived early the next morning. While Jeff asked me how I slept. I briefly thought back to the toast the nurse and I shared the night before. I told him, "All right."

The hospital has a library on the eighth floor. They not only had books to check out but also quite an assortment of movies for your viewing pleasure. The kids picked out some videos to watch. One of the ones they chose was *Bambi*, well I'm telling you it had been a long time since I watched that movie and as the story line goes the mother dies, it hit me hard. I cried. They thought it was because Bambi's mother had died. They never knew that I was crying because I started to see a correlation between the two of us.

After the movie we ate. My mother said that if you have red beans and rice to eat on New Year's Day, it would bring you good fortune the rest of the year. Believe me I would've eaten grass had she said the same about it. She made a crock-pot full of a red beans and rice concoction and we all ate it. So much for eating the traditional turkey or ham on New Year's Day! My main course from now on will be red beans and rice. We have managed to continue the tradition to this day. We still are working on

175

perfecting the recipe a bit and haven't quite got the seasonings down but let it be known it is a joyous work in progress.

The visits, whenever the family came, were always too short or so it seemed. On New Year's Day it was the same. I was excited before they got there in anticipation of their arrival, I could hardly contain myself. I would pace back and forth in my room, which was some feat considering its size. The hours flew by while we visited until they left. Then I was alone again. When I was alone I thought that the time passed by as slow as a snail. It felt like an eternity before we would see each other again.

Chapter Twenty-four

IT WASN'T TOO LONG AFTER THE New Year's Day celebration that my doctor blew into town and into my room. He made the announcement that he would let me go home and return in five days (I was in remission once again). At that time I would start the conditioning phase for the bone marrow transplant. I found out later from one of the nurses that I would be the first autologous bone marrow transplant for acute leukemia he had treated. There you have it, I always knew I had star qualities! Just as fast as he blew in, he left. If my recollection serves me right his sudden departure left me sitting there on the edge of the bed with my mouth hanging open. Even to this day when he enters a room he commands your attention and then he disappears. Flair for the dramatics, don't you think?

No one knew that home to me represented family, wellness, safety, love, warmth, people and the most important of all good cooking. Why is it that all hospitals have the worst food possible? Must be some kind of cafeteria conspiracy I think. No matter where I go and where I have stayed in the hospital the food all tastes the same, blah. I never realized you could make so many recipes from chicken. Chicken is the mainstay of any hospital cafeteria.

You don't have to twist my arm or tell me twice that I can go home before I have my bags packed. I called Jeff right away to tell him I was able to go home that day. He was as thrilled as I was until he found out it was only for five days, then he sounded disappointed. I thought five days out of this place would be like an eternity to me. All he could think about was that it wasn't enough time for us all to be together.

When he got there from home we still had to wait to be discharged. I have discovered one thing over the years, it isn't hard to get admitted to either of the hospitals in Rochester, but you play hell trying to get out. For some reason they don't want to let go. I have spent numerous hours just waiting around for someone or something so I could go home. Hmm, perhaps another conspiracy, maybe they were in cahoots with the people from food service. Do you think that sounds somewhat paranoid or what?

I made use of my time at home, I baked, cleaned and did all those wife and mom things I always thought before were boring. I would get up and spend time with the kids before they went to school and would be there when they came home. For five wonderful glorious days we were living like normal once again. I went to do some visiting before I was shut up again. I went to the floor and saw all my nurse comrades. Then I went back to the nursing school I graduated from to see my instructors. Being the extrovert I am this was good for my ego just like a preverbal shot in the arm.

The five days flew by so fast it felt as though I had just blinked my eyes and poof I was gone. Before I took a breath we were on our way through the back roads of Iowa and Minnesota in the darkness of the early morning to check into the hospital for my transplant. Adventurous, aren't I? Not at all. Scared stiff? You bet! I have found that until I have experienced something once I panic more, but when I have gone through some new experience I relax some. Now I didn't say totally, I said some. I didn't sleep the night before; I find to this day I don't always sleep well before a checkup.

After we checked in I was once again escorted to the BMT unit. Jeff and I walked in following the escort. Much to my surprise I was given a much larger room than I had five days before. They still weren't done with the renovation of the old BMT unit, so we had to go back to the temporary unit. The view from my window still wasn't the greatest and I couldn't watch my geese I had become attached to. No exercise cycle either, but it was definitely one room I could move around in.

We measured the length of the room from my bed to the door and calculated how many times I would have to walk back and forth to equal a mile. I was all pumped up to keep myself in shape during my time of being shut up, wasn't I? I was being quite optimistic, even with my optimism I was not able to keep it up when my blood counts hit rock bottom. I was ready to win one for the gipper, which deserves an "E" for the effort. Who was the gipper? I remember that it was something coaches always said to get their team to get them pumped up to win a game. I was gearing up for my game too; one I had every intention of winning.

The same day I checked in I also started my chemotherapy. I was to receive two different types of chemotherapy during this conditioning phase. The goal was to totally destroy the bone marrow I had presently, clearing the way for new marrow to replace it. Normally, they use total body radiation in place of one of the types of chemotherapy. Instead my doctor decided to go with Busulfan, a chemotherapy agent, in place of the radiation. It had the same effect as radiation, even to the degree that my skin turned a brownish color. I think if you want a tan though you should still go outdoors or go to a tanning salon, don't try radiation it's expensive and isn't good for you.

I found it fascinating, I also thought if they could throw some sand around on my hospital room floor, along with some seashells I could send everyone a picture and let them think I was really on a beach in Florida. Hey, if you get a tan at the prices I

179

was paying, let's put it to good use is how I figured it. Who cares if it's artificial or not?

The one drawback of Busulfan is that I had to take four huge capsules every six hours round the clock; they even would wake me in the night to give them to me. Inside these capsules (which were clear) were ten little pills. The pharmacy put the pills in the capsules to help patients take them. Otherwise could you imagine swallowing forty pills every six hours, regardless if they were tiny, no one could do that for very long. I hate taking pills anyway so anything that made it easier for the medicine to go down was a godsend to me. I often wondered if a spoonful of sugar would have helped the medicine go down.

After I finished the days of pills, I received intravenous chemotherapy through my Hickman. The drug was called Cytoxan; this was powerful stuff. I needed to have a catheter placed in my bladder; as well as be hooked up to a heart monitor for the two days I received it. Nasty stuff. They kept me somewhat sedated through the infusion too, because it had a tendency to make you really sick so they loaded me up as a preventative measure. Once all the chemotherapy was completed I had what they called a day of rest. It was a day where they sort of left me alone, no drugs of any kind. Ahhhh! A day of rest from vomiting and nausea was great. This stuff truly was one of the worst for side effects.

Finally the day! January 23, 1990, came for the actual transplant. Hooray, we made it! Jeff took the day off from work to be with me. We felt that this was the beginning of a new life together, and we wanted to share it with each other.

I was surprised to see how the transplant was done. In my own uninformed mind I thought it was some big deal to have them perform this. Not really, the marrow comes in a small bag just like blood does, only it isn't as red, it's a sort of pinkish-yellow color. They administer it just like a transfusion too, once they thawed it outside my room. Bone marrow is stored with your name and record number on it, so when needed they just thaw it. It is stored in a preservative called DMSO that I told you about earlier. But what I didn't tell you is that it smells like garlic when the body tries to rid itself of it through your pores. I've reached new heights! I've gone from getting a fake tan to smelling like a salad. It's a great combo to keep the vampires at bay. Oh, the wonders of modern chemistry; it's grand, isn't it?

The transplant process was all new to us and we discovered we had a lot to learn. The nurses were really good about making sure we were kept informed. The restrictions afterwards were the worst. No fresh vegetables or fruits for three months. All my meat had to be well done, that is really hard for me, I enjoy my prime rib rare. I couldn't be around pets, this was bad because we had two dogs, two cats, and a bird named Jake. We had to farm them out for six months. My mother took one of the dogs, our close neighbors took one of the cats, and the rest went to different friends' homes. I couldn't have any household plants or work in the garden outdoors. This was going to really suck I thought.

When the bone marrow was administered I was sedated, and again placed on a heart monitor. When it was done infusing and bringing me new life everyone simply packed up their stuff and went away. The way I thought, I was expecting the crescendo of music from the *2001 Space Odyssey* movie from the seventies to be playing. But nothing, so I played it in my head for myself. While I was in the US Navy I expected the same music should be played when there was a birth of a baby. There are just some things that warrant that music, and this was one of them…

After the transplant was complete we returned to the all familiar waiting game, this I was used to. I don't do the waiting very well but I'm trying. I must say that I was not blessed with a whole lot of patience. Sometimes I think that keeping me waiting like they did was a way to perhaps make me more patient. Well it didn't work.

This time I was the sickest I had ever been, not just nausea, vomiting and diarrhea, which I did plenty of, but mouth sores that made it difficult to swallow my own saliva. I had to be put on a morphine drip again. I had to use a handheld suction device to help suck up my spit. I also was experiencing dizziness. Every time I picked my head up off the pillow the room would start to spin. Not a good feeling believe me.

I couldn't eat; every time I did I would bring it back up. I stuck to a lot of Jell-O, I remember the diet tech telling me to keep in mind what goes down usually comes back up so don't eat anything too heavy. To this day I cannot eat peach Jell-O; in fact, I shudder at the thought of it.

Many fevers brought lots of antibiotics. What do they say, sometimes the cure can be worse than the disease? I know this isn't true because without the transplant I would've died, I was fighting hard to keep from dying during this rescue. But when you are really sick, you sometimes don't think there will be an end to it all, let alone save you.

Chapter Twenty-five

JEFF AND MY MOM WOULD ALTERNATE coming up to see me. They both had jobs and so they shared the responsibility of trying to keep my spirits up. It wasn't easy for them either; it was winter so the roads could be treacherous. One Saturday, when I was really in rough shape, Jeff came to see me. He had been working at home after work installing a shower in the bathroom off of our bedroom. We had a shower but it was in the basement, he knew I wouldn't be able to maneuver the stairs so he did the next best thing, put a shower upstairs. It was great! Anyway while he visited me that day I was so sick that he went home and told my mother he couldn't go up the next day. He says now that he truly felt that he wouldn't be taking me home at all. It scared him so much he was avoiding having to see me.

It was funny when my mom came to sit with me that next day, a sunny Sunday morning. Mom sat by the window reading her Sunday paper while I slept. The warmth of the sun made the room toasty. The consultant on the transplant service walked into my room leading the rest of his entourage, asking me when I wanted to go home. I sat upright in bed and answered him with a strong reply, "Wednesday." Seeing as this was Sunday, it meant in three days I would be walking out of there.

My mother was shocked; she couldn't believe that they were actually going to release me. All I needed was to recuperate; the hard part was over. I felt, as did the doctors, I would do that better at home. It was the isolation that was getting to me the most. We called Jeff; he couldn't believe his ears. From what I looked like to him the day before, gave him no indication that I would be well enough to leave the hospital ever, let alone in three days. I needed to have contact with my people again.

Believe it or not I did get out of the hospital on that Wednesday. The only problem was I couldn't go all the way home right away. I was to stay some place in Rochester, because I had to go to the clinic every day to check my blood counts and be seen by the doctor. My mother was going to stay with me; she took a week off from work to stay with me in Rochester. Jeff was running short of vacation days.

We first went to the transplant house as a possible choice to stay but found out that we were going to have to help clean and cook. Jeff opted to put us up in a hotel in the downtown area. My mother was in her fifties, not old by any means, but she has had a terrible car accident in her younger years and even though she is not disabled she didn't need to be cleaning as well as taking care of me. As for me, well I could barely walk, my feet were so swollen they didn't even fit in shoes, I had to wear slippers. I remember my first night in the hotel; my mother helped me take a bath, as she washed my back I started to cry. All I thought of was that this whole thing sucked big time! At least I wasn't in the hospital though, hooray for that! I did have to wear a mask at all times whenever I was out in public. It was a heavy mask and at times I felt like I sounded like Darth Vader trying to breathe.

My daily challenge was to walk through the subway system below the clinic buildings from our hotel to have my tests done. Thank goodness there were little benches along the route that resembled jump seats the stewardesses sat in on a plane during takeoffs and landings. We'd walk about forty feet, sit for twenty minutes then walk again. It took quite awhile to reach our destination. Each day got a little bit easier, I could walk further and further between rests.

We stayed in the hotel for five days; things are pretty sketchy during the time. It must be the drugs! After the five days I was able to go all the way home, with a scheduled return appointment for one week. Sleeping in my own bed felt great! I still had some residual nausea, vomiting, and diarrhea, but I seemed none the worse for wear.

Weakness still prevailed, yet my mother would make me put my winter coat on every day, along with my slippers and begin the process of regaining my strength by walking. I can remember just walking two houses from ours down the street to the corner and crying because my feet hurt so bad. I was frustrated, I wanted to have it all back, to be strong again and I wanted it now. Remember what I said about patience? This must be another test.

My mother told me at that time I needed to be patient that even as a child you have to go to kindergarten before you can go to first grade, this was my kindergarten. And an infant must crawl before they can walk. This was my crawling and kindergarten stage. That soothed my emotional pain for the time, I knew she was right, one step at a time and I would eventually be back in the swing of things.

Whenever we went to the clinic for an appointment after the blood draw at seven o'clock in the morning we would get something to eat and go to the mall. Why? I didn't have an appointment until three-thirty in the afternoon.

When we got back to the clinic we would people watch; some interesting things took place. First, we noticed that most people would walk way around me because I had a scarf and mask on. They didn't understand that I needed the protection from them. We also watched an older couple who had their glasses slide off their noses and hang by one earpiece. The last thing was Jeff being the prankster he is, he would go to the middle of the room and stare up at the skylight for a short while. When he returned to his seat we waited to see how long it would take before someone went over to check out what he had been looking at. He was always trying to *make me laugh*! All we could do was to try to muffle our laughing as best we could.

My checkups went well. Each visit I asked my doctor when I could have vegetables and fruits. It was driving me crazy, naturally when you are told you can't have something that is all you crave. Well the same held true in this instance, I was craving salads, apples, bananas, corn anything that I couldn't have. I felt like one of Pavlov's dogs, I would find myself salivating at the sight of lettuce or tomatoes.

It was three months before I was allowed to have fruits with thick skins. Melons were something I liked to eat and could have. I nearly was on a food binge eating so much of them. This probably amounted to about one half cup at each meal, if I could keep it down. I called it binge eating! This relieved some of my cravings, but only momentarily. It wasn't long after that I was allowed to have anything with a peel or skin. By June 1, I was pretty much eating most things, and believe it or not the cravings went away.

My strength came back faster once my feet were no longer swollen. I was able to go for long walks, as well as go up and down stairs. The beginning of my new life was slowly coming back to me. When my doctor finally told me to arrange at home to have my Hickman removed I knew I was all right. I had one of the surgeons I knew from work remove the Hickman. Hooray, now there weren't many telltale signs left of the ordeal. Nothing like the first time when, after the Hickman was removed, my entire left breast was one giant bruise.

In August of 1990 I was able to jump the last hurdle, I got to have my dogs and cats back plus I was able to return to work. Amen! I was nervous my first day back because I still didn't have any hair and I wouldn't go anywhere without my head covered so I needed scarves that I could wear with my uniforms. It wouldn't be for long though once I went back to work that I was able to uncover my head showing my new growth of one half inch of almost black hair. I think I felt a little like Dorothy from the

Wizard of Oz, who always said, "There's no place like home!" Ain't it the truth!

I no longer believe that leukemia or cancer in general is a disaster. My I have grown over the years. Not, if you ask my children though, they accuse me of still being a child. *Nothing wrong with that*, I thought. I still enjoy cracking jokes, laughing, pulling pranks, giggling in church when I read a wrong word while we were supposed to be singing. My daughter always egged me on by laughing at me. My son told me I sure don't act like other moms my age.

Stress, the silent but deadly killer, sneaks up on you. When you least expect it, you are suddenly plagued with a cold, headache, or backache. Sometimes it can be more severe, heart attacks, ulcers or even cancer. I could go on but I think you get the picture. From what I could see I was under stress. That's one theory I believe contributes to our illnesses—especially cancer.

That warm feeling we all get when adrenaline starts activating the fight or flight response, worked well on our ancestors the caveman. They needed to either run like hell from the dinosaurs or stop, kill and eat them or become their dinner. But when all of their muscles tensed up they were able to release that tension in order to fight to survive.

Nowadays, engaging the need to fight or flee only puts undue stress on our bodies. It starts the flow of many different natural chemicals, which are dumped into the system. We no longer have to fight for our safety on a regular basis just to go to sleep at night. So what happens now is that we internalize things, so this is a tearing down of our own body giving way for illnesses to take over—cancer, ulcers, heart disease, heart attacks or just a general feeling like crap.

Negativity is one thought I truly couldn't afford to have both then and now. Negativity breeds negativity. Negative thinking doesn't give you a life-threatening or any other kind of illness, it simply produces the opportunity. It wears you down, depleting your body's own immune system, you are now primed and ready for illness to set in.

Chapter Twenty-six

EVERY DAY AND EVERYWHERE YOU GO in life you can overhear someone say, "That's not normal." I have often wondered who decides what is normal and what is not. Normal according to *Webster's Dictionary* states that, "*conforming to with accepted standard or norm; natural; usual.*" And the definition of norm is "*a standard or model.*" I say that what is normal for me and what is normal for you is the truth behind normalcy. I don't think that anyone truly knows what the definition of normal is.

Needless to say my family returned to their normal lives. Each of us going in different directions: swimming, running, eating, working, studying, walking and even arguing at times. But this was normal for us and we loved it. We all kind of relaxed a bit. Rarely did we talk about all we went through, looking back we felt this would not enable us to go forward. Why dwell on it, it was for all practical purposes over with. We were really good about denying the events even took place.

When teenagers turn into young adults, I'm not sure when this happens but it does, they seem to leave the nest more often. Much to the chagrin of their parents, who still view them at the age they were when they taught them to look both ways before crossing a street. Crossing the street was easy to learn, it is the other things they encounter in their daily lives that aren't as easy. We wanted to protect them, only to find we were trying to control them.

We had always taught our children to be independent thinkers. To take a stand for what is right or for something they believed in. I didn't realize that it also meant they could stand up to their parents, oddly enough that meant Jeff and I, it was a form of rebellion. Don't get me wrong they are wonderful children and I wouldn't change anything about them, but it was hard to believe that they would challenge us from time to time. You know typical teens and we fell into the trap of being typical parents.

When the children entered high school we made a pact with them, if they could go through all four years without smoking, drinking or drugs, on graduation day we would give them one thousand dollars. Their grandmother made them the same deal. So what this meant was on the date they received their diploma they would receive two thousand dollars. Pretty good deal I thought. Would I have been able to do that at eighteen, nah? Was it bribery, you bet! In the time we live in, when children are killing other children, we thought if we could keep the other things out of their hands they would at least have a fighting chance out there.

Children in the new millennium have harder times then children in my generation. Everything is so technological now, back then it was a big deal to have television and if you had two you were considered to be wealthy. Now it's computers, everyone has them; it is becoming almost impossible to get along without them. There are people who don't want to learn about them and bury their heads in the sand letting the world pass them by. In our family alone we have three of the things. Why? Well each of the kids needed a computer when they went to college and with Jeff in the computer arena he could get them reasonable deals. Besides he could also fix any problems they might have.

The children of today are bombarded with video games,

movies, VCRs, Game Boys, computers, the Internet, CD players, yet they still came to their father and I telling us how bored they were. On a lazy summer day when I was young, I can remember lying in the back yard on the grass and looking up at the sky to see what things I could make from the clouds, dogs, cats, dinosaurs, teddy bears or just waves rolling along. Not a care in the world. Not anymore, they want you to entertain them. Oh, how I long for the good life, in simpler times!

The children of the new millennium believe that they need to be entertained. Their imaginations have been dulled, their senses are not as keen, and they are becoming robots. This to me is ironic after seeing the movie *Bicentennial Man*, where the story line had to do with a robot that wanted to be human. Perhaps we are somewhat backwards.

I believe that children should be children and not miniature adults; they will get there all too soon. I guess that is enough soap boxing for now. Remember I did tell you that in our family we stand up for what we believe in. This is not a book on parenting even though sometimes raising your little bundles of joy would be easier if they only came with manuals at birth.

After I returned from the hospital and my bone marrow transplant I was as weak as a kitten. I needed help showering, getting dressed, cutting my food and walking. I don't do the helpless thing real well, which led to many more hours and days of frustration. Let's put all the cards on the table, I don't handle change well either. Having someone doing my cleaning, cooking, laundry I had enjoyed before I got sick. Now, it drove me through the roof, I wanted to do it all myself...I was not used to having to ask my children to help me dress in the morning or have to have someone in the house before I could take a shower for fear I was too weak to be left alone to do this.

I was on a mission to return to my life, the comfortable routine I had established through the years. This I found was my greatest motivation in the world. I knew I had to get moving and take back my home. This doesn't mean I didn't appreciate all the help I received from family and friends because I did.

There is absolutely no way to ever repay the kindness,

generosity, love and support I received. People are wonderful!

That is why we have continued our annual pig roasts, as a way of saying thank you. It became more than a thank you, it turned into more of a celebration of life. It has mushroomed over the years though; we started with maybe a meager fifty people attending and have now reached one hundred and fifty. I always say let's party!

We decided that we needed more family time. That instead of always being jealous of those families that took vacations together each year, we needed to become one of them. In the fall of 1990 we took our first family vacation, we went to visit Grandma and Grandpa in Maine (Jeff's parents). It was Thanksgiving; we had an absolutely wonderful time.

We promised that in four years we would return for another visit. I've always been disappointed that our children have never spent more time with their other set of grandparents. Being the ages the kids were, Justin ten, and Jennifer nearly thirteen, they didn't want to spend all their vacations in Maine. They wanted to do kid things; you know what they called "fun." That is why we said we would be back in four years; it was sort of a compromise.

In January of 1991 Jeff and I took a four-day trip to Las Vegas. This was the first anniversary of my bone marrow transplant. We wanted to be together to celebrate the start of our new life together. Thinking back on it now, perhaps it was a little selfish of us to not include the children in our celebration. They always say that hindsight is twenty-twenty.

What we did learn from the experience is that it is good to get away. Things become a little clearer and we are better able to handle the stress when we have had some playtime. I had always heard that it was important to have playtime as a child, but why only as a child? What that basically says is that we let the children have all the fun. This is definitely a bad idea. They even have recess as part of the curriculum when you are in elementary school. I just want to say, take me back to kindergarten.

Perhaps there should be recess throughout all of the school years, kindergarten through twelfth. It may sound strange but if it were what might be considered normal, knowing nothing different, we could eliminate some of the problems that teens encounter as they get older. I have read somewhere that exercise; a lot of laughter as well as being allowed to play are good for you. So, let's just think of it like this; if you can laugh while you exercise playing volleyball, does that help you to understand it now? This means that if you get the formula right healing can begin.

Some of us need to teach ourselves how to play, to let out the inner child. Recess at work might be a good suggestion, what do you think? I find that having time to play as well as work makes a much more rounded person. To get away from the drudgery and stress of our lives for even a short time can make things a lot better. It changes your mental attitude, your outlook on life. Our family has found that you don't have to go through the extravagance of traveling to far off destinations to have a fun vacation. We have taken day trips in our own state, to go to fairs, hobo days and even buffalo days and had the best fun and relaxation ever. We are together and spending time away from the normal routine.

Oftentimes when money is tight I will go to a card shop just to read the humorous cards. It can be kind of embarrassing being the only bald person in the store, practically rolling in the aisles after reading something that tickles my funny bones. I just think that they are ones that have lost touch with their child within. Don't shut he or she out, let them out to teach you how to play again. Remember we use fewer muscles to smile than frown.

Try this little test, the next time you are walking into work, a store or just out for a stroll. When you encounter someone along the way smile at them, if you are feeling brave that day then say good morning. I have recently started looking at names on the person's nametag and when I leave their presence, albeit restaurant or grocery store, I tell them "thank you" adding their name. I can guarantee you that you will feel much better and you may have made a difference in the persons you met on your way. Keep in mind; they always say that there are no strangers in the world just friends you haven't met yet!

Chapter Twenty-seven

THE FOLLOWING YEAR WE PLANNED THAT long awaited fun-filled vacation. When the kids got out of school we flew to Florida and spent a week at Disney World. The kids had so much fun I couldn't believe it, Justin on occasion would complain about his sore feet (he still to this day complains about his feet being sore after he gets off work). In spite of that, we sure had fun!

We rented a minivan for the week we were in Orlando. We came and went whenever we wanted. Our hotel had three swimming pools so in the mornings the kids swam. And in the late afternoon we would head to the Disney World parks. We discovered that everyone enjoyed themselves more if we rested at the hotel during the hottest part of the day, going to the parks for evening activities. It made a lot more sense than hauling the kids to the parks ordering them to have fun as I lathered them with sunscreen in preparation for temperatures in the eighties and sometimes nineties.

We always went to get something good to eat; the kid's favorite was the Olive Garden, not McDonald's or Burger King either. Then we would pack our backpack with snacks like apples, crackers and fruit drinks. After our first visit to the park concession stand, spending over twelve dollars on three lemonades, we figured out that it was too rich for our taste to be eating while we played.

In our hotel room we had a microwave and a small refrigerator. This made it easy to keep milk and whatever else we needed to keep cold. So the kids were able to have their breakfast in our room, all we needed was the cereal. Our hotel did not have a breakfast for the guests, nowadays, most of the hotels serve continental breakfasts where there is a big selection of foods including waffles.

Having our own vehicle enabled us to have more freedom. We even drove down to see my uncle who lives near Fort Meyers, in the town of Cape Coral. We spent a whole day with him and his wife. It had been several years since I had seen either of them. Having their own pool gave Jennifer and Justin another opportunity to paddle around in the water. We grilled steaks and had a super time just being together and getting to know my uncle and aunt all over again.

When I was younger I didn't realize how important having family ties were. I pretty much went out into the world all on my own, barely having contact with my own mother. So being able to spend time with my uncle was great. Jeff comes from a large family and the family ties are strong, so that whenever he comes home to visit we are usually inundated with family.

How I longed for those types of family relationships. I think my daughter does too. She is getting married in two thousand one and her fiancé has extended family connections like my husband did. We have extended family living in our town and don't have get-togethers or contact at all with about half of them. I think she would like to have better communication with her family, but feels that at this time it is impossible.

To call my family (not my immediate family mind you) dysfunctional is an understatement. I often think it would be nice if everyone could forget their petty jealousies and differences to share some quality family time with one another. I doubt if I'll ever see it come to pass. Oh well I guess it's all our loss.

Suffering from a life crisis like I did gives one time to think how stupid most family disagreements are. Everyone is too proud to say I'm sorry, that is the downfall of most relationships. What is truly going to be sad is if anything happens to one of them, which is a time that family regrets the loss of contact they could've had.

The time we shared together as a family after my transplant was wonderful. Not only was it normal, it was peaceful, happy and loving. Even though I was back at work, we tried to not let the children become latchkey children. Jeff worked from seven until four Monday through Friday. I worked from three until eleven with varying days off. The kids spent only one hour a day without supervision.

Until they were in fifth grade they always went to our sitter, which was like going home for them. We were really blessed finding a sitter like we had; I smile to myself when I hear of friends talking about having childcare problems. Once they were in fifth grade they were given a house key that they wore around their necks on florescent orange shoelaces. The rules were that no one was allowed to come over to visit, and they couldn't go anywhere until their dad came home from work. The time was supposed to be spent doing homework, so that when Dad came home they could go outdoors once he checked things out with them from their day.

When I went back to work I would often call home in the evenings to check on how everything was going, only to discover that it was eight o'clock and no one had eaten yet. If you asked Mr. Marsters why they hadn't eaten it was because the kids were outside playing and didn't want to come in to eat. If you ask the kids it was because Dad was too busy to fix them supper.

My husband loves the outdoors growing everything he can get his hands on. Then the rest of the time he works hard to take care of it all. Regardless, I took charge and started making the meals during the day with specific instructions on what to do to finish off the meal. Things worked out quite well after that. It's not that he can't cook, it's that the kids being kids just didn't always like his choices for meals. That's not to say that they have always given me the thumbs up on my cooking either, the odds were better with me though. I would make something they liked.

One of their father's favorite meals is Spam and beans, well five nights a week is a bit much. Justin to this day won't eat beans. Jennifer, on the other hand, is definitely her father's daughter; she loves them. It's nothing for those two to cook up a pot of the stuff together then sit down and consume it all.

The summer of 1993 brought with it yet another family vacation, this time to the other coast, the old California or bust. Jeff's sister and her husband lived in Santa Barbara, so we went for a visit. After we arrived we packed up our rental car, bringing along Jeff's sister and headed for the mountains. We went to Yosemite and Sequoia National Parks. The most beautiful things I had ever seen. Naturally the kids weren't as excited about the scenery as Jeff and I were. Justin was just as happy sitting in the front seat playing with all the bells and whistles the rental car had on it.

Jennifer would have been much happier if we would have just dropped her off at some mall. This is funny to her father and I now because her fiancé is quite the outdoorsman. Now Jennifer thinks camping in near primitive conditions, hiking and backpacking are the best activities in the world. Had we suggested this when she was sixteen all we would have gotten was a long moan.

Driving through the backcountry of California and then down the coastal highway from San Francisco back to Santa Barbara we logged seventeen hundred miles in four days. We then spent two days with Jeff's sister before heading for the grand finale, Disneyland. We had made reservations at the Disneyland hotel and also to have breakfast the next morning with Mickey and the gang. It was wonderful, but just like all other vacations we have taken it wasn't long before we had to head home. What is the phrase, all good things must come to an end. And so it did. Back home, back to reality. Even though you may never get the kids to admit it, they were changed by the experience. We all were amazed at the beauty of this country we live in, and this will stay with us for the rest of our lives.

All of the vacations, along with work and household chores, were quite successful in helping me put out of my mind the fact that I had cancer. You know the old out of sight out of mind sort of thing. I could at least put it out of my mind until I would get the envelope in the mail. The envelope with all of the little folders in it telling me where to go and what to do in preparation of my next visit to Rochester. This was when it always came flooding back to me. Even today I can get myself revved up before I head to Rochester for a checkup. I use Pavlov's conditioning theory as a reference. I hear or see Rochester I don't salivate like Pavlov's dogs, I palpitate.

Chapter Twenty-eight

WE WERE GETTING READY FOR OUR trip to Maine in March of 1994. Remember I said that we were going to go see Jeff's family every four years; well it had been four years. We had four years of kid vacations and now it was time for adult vacations. The end of March the children had a week of spring break off from school so that is when we decided to leave.

During this time we were also housing a foreign exchange student from the Netherlands. She had come to live with us the August before. She spoke English very well. The only problem was that she wasn't very motivated to participate in family activities. She was a competitive swimmer, so in school she was allowed to swim on the varsity squad as a senior. While we would be heading to Maine she opted to go to New York City with her exchange group for spring break, which was fine with us. We knew that for her, it was an opportunity of a lifetime.

It was Friday night, and I started my vacation the next day, so I was pretty upbeat at the desk that evening. The census was fairly low so we had some downtime to laugh and chat around the nurse's station. I remember calling Jeff at home trying to convince him to come in and take a break with me. I was using all kinds of funny stuff just to see if he would give in, but no he said that he was going to relax, he was on vacation. We were to fly to Maine out of Minneapolis the following Tuesday.

At around ten-thirty one of the nurses stepped out of a patient's room and into the hallway announcing that we needed to "Call a code." Whenever we had a Code 4 (cardiac arrest) on the unit the adrenaline rush is there to spur you into action. So naturally being the charge nurse I ran to the room to help. Shortly the code team arrived and at this time each crash cart (the main cart used for medication administration, intubations, defibrillation, plus a whole lot more) was not the same on each floor so the code team had to rummage through the drawers trying to find the items they needed. I was being the good gopher and went to the clean utility room for things the code team thought wasn't on or in the crash cart.

The increase of adrenaline in my system, coupled with an undiagnosed cardiomyopathy (causing irregular heartbeats) put me into ventricular fibrillation (V-fib). This meant I was in full cardiac arrest; they had to call a second code for me. Two codes at the same time, on the same floor and in the evening was almost too much for everyone there to handle.

I had run to the clean utility room for something the code team wanted. As I pushed open the door and stepped in; I put one foot through the door and fell back into a coworker's arms. She had followed me to help me locate the items needed.

Today wherever I go in the Mayo Clinic system and tell them about my experience I always hear "so you're the one." There, I am infamous.

The evening supervisor called Jeff at home, trying to tell him that I needed him and he should come right away. They couldn't convince him that it was not a joke. He thought I had put her up to calling him to come in for a break. She finally had to put a friend of mine on the phone who was crying and she finally convinced him this was not a joke and something serious was going on. He came right away, when he finally realized they were all telling him the truth. At that time I was still arresting.

When Jeff arrived I was still down in the clean utility and they were working on me. By then the whole gang was all there: Vice President, Director of Nursing, my head nurse, supervisors, chaplains, doctors and nurses galore. When they announce a cardiac arrest over the PA system they always give the location, when the staff who were working throughout the hospital that evening heard that there was a cardiac arrest in the clean utility room they knew it had to be a staff person involved. The utility rooms, clean or dirty, are off-limits to patients. Even though they figured it was a staff member they just didn't know who it could be.

I have read the book *Embraced by the Light* about one woman's experiencing what happens when you die. Well I can't tell you I saw any lights. But I can tell you I heard them all calling my name. "Come on, Jeanine," they were yelling. All I remember is feeling a sense of peace and calm. My response in my mind to their insistence I come back is that I would get there when I was ready, not to rush me. So whatever I saw or heard or sensed was something that I wasn't all that ready to give up. After thirty minutes they were able to get my heart back in a normal sinus rhythm.

I was then transported to the CCU where I remained on a ventilator and asleep for three days. When they first got me up there and into bed I was "bucking the vent," a phrase used by nursing personnel for someone that is quite restless and thrashing about while on the ventilator. It was at that point that the doctor that took charge of my case decided to put me to sleep. I was given a medication that would sedate me and keep me under until he deemed it was a good time to wake me up.

During that time I was taken for CT scans, had EEGs and multiple blood tests. They wanted to determine if there had been any brain damage, heart damage or anything that would not return me to a normal life. Then everyone waited, the nurses, the doctors and my family. All who knew me waited and watched to see what was going to happen next. Jeff spent most of the time at the hospital in the waiting room, where all our friends who were concerned about me visited him. The kids were doing okay, but Jennifer lingered back and would not come in to see me on the ventilator. She just couldn't she said. She didn't want to see me like that.

Jennifer was the only one that kept asking everybody about my contact lenses. She knew I was still wearing them! She couldn't convince anyone because no one was listening. So when they were about to wake me up, guess what they found? You got it; I still had the contacts in. Once they removed them, Jennifer's response was, "No one ever listens to the kid!"

Jeff told my doctor that he wanted to be in the room when the doctor woke me up, because he thought I would freak out thinking that it was something to do with my leukemia returning. So there he was leaning over the side rails of the bed and yelling to me that I was all right, that it wasn't my leukemia returning I just had a "small problem with my heart."

I motioned to him that I wanted to write something by waving my arm in the air. Seeing as I couldn't talk with the tube in my throat, he gave me a clipboard with a sheet of paper on it and a pencil. No one knew what my response was going to be. I wrote down, "You call this small!" He started laughing the first sound of laughter he made since I arrested. He said that it was then that he knew I was back and that I was myself, that I was NORMAL. Again I ask, what is normal, normal for my family is making it through one crisis at a time. The one thing I can say that is truly normal for me is that I do know how to have fun and you should see my collection of coloring books and crayons!

Chapter Twenty-nine

TO THIS DAY I FIND IT hard to believe that my heart actually stopped beating. I was considered clinically dead! It stills gives me goose bumps when I think back on what happened. I wanted to know why this was happening to me at all. I asked everyone, including God. No one was sure, but assured me they would get to the bottom of it.

Even though our heart center at the hospital is good and up to date, they still don't have an electrophysiology department, (where they can check the electrical functioning of the heart) which is what I needed. I was still doped up on medication so they asked Jeff where he wanted me to be transferred; his choices were Des Moines or Rochester. (And because I was conditioned by Pavlov to balk at the idea of Rochester, I was opting for Des Moines.) Thank goodness no one listened to me, except the doctor who wanted me to go to Des Moines too.

The doctor and Jeff had a small go around as the arrangements were being made. The doctor tried to tell him that it was my choice to go to Des Moines. Jeff explained that if I wasn't affected by the medications that I would choose Rochester over Des Moines with no questions asked. They had saved my life before and Jeff had every confidence in the staff there. He won; I was to be transferred to Rochester.

Before I left they wanted to do a cardiac catherization, which would check out my heart a little closer. Jeff again spoke up and told them that they would only repeat the test in Rochester. Unless it would alter my condition or treatment in some way, he insisted they not do it. He won that round too. I'm sure they were happy to transfer me anywhere just as long as it was out of there.

I don't remember much about the ambulance ride up there other than the gurneys they use for transporting patients are not comfortable for anything other than going around the block. But I guess most of the time their passengers are unconscious and comfortable sleeping arrangements were the least of their worries.

When I arrived at Rochester St. Mary's Hospital I was admitted to a cardiac step-down unit, and put on telemetry. (This is a system that is used to allow the staff to watch the patient's heart rhythm without having to run EKG strips all the time. (Telemetry is like a continuous EKG.) The monitors were being watched in a central station, located on the unit, by trained personnel.

Next, a cardiologist, followed by an electrophysiologist visited me. I was run through about every test they could think of to determine what caused the incident, including a cardiac catheterization. They pretty much had it figured out by learning about my history. One of the chemotherapy agents I was given has cardiac side effects, arrhythmias (abnormal heart rhythms) being one of them. I didn't know that it was a possibility and I am a nurse. In my own defense though I am not a cardiac or oncology nurse, I'm a surgical nurse. The doctors cut on them, we get them up and running again.

In the electrophysiology department they actually put me into V-fib. If the rhythm could be induced while being tested then they would move on to the next step. The next step would be implantation of an ICD (internal cardiac defibrillator). They would implant this as well as the leads that attached to it so if I would go into V-fib at any time the device would give me the necessary shock or shocks needed to convert me to a normal heart rhythm.

This is what happens in external defibrillation; now this gizmo would enable my heart do this itself. I wondered if it ran on Eveready or Duracell batteries. Just the pink bunny and I, we keep on going and going and going...I could do a whole comedy routine regarding the little wonder. To start things off I named him Chester; how fitting, don't you think? Chester and I were very close; in fact, you could say he was especially close to my heart. To this day Jeff thinks I am luckier than anyone else, because he thinks that everyone doesn't have a Chester to lookout at all times for something to go wrong. He says he is kind of jealous.

The day before they put the leads into my heart I went into an abnormal rhythm called V-tach, which simply means that my ventricles were beating faster then the rest of my heart. They had to start medication to change the rhythm back, believe me this didn't do much for my emotional state. I was scared out of my mind anyway so all this did was keep me there.

Jeff stayed in Rochester the whole time I was there. I was able to watch him walk to his hotel at the end of the day and he would stop, look up and wave to me as he headed for sleep. I didn't feel as alone as I did in past hospitalizations. I believe from all those times he spent sitting next to my bed over the years has succeeded in one thing; he has become very restless.

He can't seem to sit still. In fact, he'll say to me when he comes in from outdoors that he is done for the day. That lasts about five minutes and he will think of something he needs to do. I, on the other hand, sat or lay in bed soooooooo much over the years that it has conformed me into a slug at times. I am perfectly content to sit and listen to music or read or do needlework. Just as long as it isn't in a hospital room setting. Don't get me wrong, I think that exercise is an important part in our lives; I just mean that I can be content now, instead of running in circles like I used to do.

They did have difficulty putting the leads to my heart, it was from all the scar tissue I now have on the left side of my chest from Hickman catheters I have had in the past. They attempted on the left anyway, not knowing they would run into scar tissue and had to finally settle for right-sided access. The device itself was put into my abdomen. It was roughly the size of a man's wallet. I spent one night in the ICU unit after they hooked me all up and then I was transferred to another step-down unit for two days and then finally home. I only needed a few weeks of recuperation after the placement of Chester before I would go back to work.

Jennifer was very vocal about her anger regarding the incident. As she put it, "I've had just about enough out of you!" I guess you could say that she wasn't too happy about my latest escapade. I think at that time she perhaps thought I enjoyed scaring the you know what out of all of them as well as myself. This wasn't true.

Justin, on the other hand, seemed to be handling it better, he was quiet and as I found out later his silence was actually deafening. He would always get up and leave the room whenever the conversation would roll around to my health. I should've taken this as a sign of a volcano starting to rumble. But as usual I had my parental blinders on.

When I left the hospital they gave me a pamphlet titled, *"The Rhythm of Life."* How appropriate, don't you think? It told about the do's and don'ts of my new life. No hot tubs, no riding horses, I couldn't even wear constricting pants around my waist. Hello polyester, knit pants? I don't think so! Once you move to those pants the next step is usually sensible shoes. As for riding horses I haven't ridden in years anyway, so I could live without it. But the hot tub seemed to put a kibosh on my social life.

One of the nurses who was going to school going for her registered nurse degree switched to the evening shift so she could go to classes during the day. She had a terrific hot tub and after a hellacious evening at work a few of us would pack up our suits and go over for some relaxation, wine and cheese. What a perfect end to a not so perfect day.

One other restriction was that I couldn't drive. Why? Because

I had a seizure during the arrest, and anyone that has had a seizure will have a driving restriction for at least six months. Naturally, I always thought I had to go someplace. What a pain, not being able to just get up and go. There were more restrictions but not any that stick out in my mind or that I objected to as much as these.

One more time it was hi-ho hi-ho, it's off to work I go. The staff on my unit was more nervous about my return than I was. But then again for the first few weeks after I returned I was working on the new employee orientation manual, so my days were uneventful. It was a nice way to ease back into the work. When I returned to my real job and my real shift then the fun began.

The first time I went to the clean utility room where the arrest happened, I could feel myself hyperventilating. I was experiencing a panic attack. The first day I was left in charge of the floor and the shift, I started panicking so my heart started racing. The evening supervisor sent me home. This was all so new to us; we were treading on unfamiliar ground. I had to force myself to go over each of these hurdles I encountered one at a time.

The first time that we had a cardiac arrest on our floor, I could feel myself getting revved up. When just about everyone in the hospital that knew my story and responded to the call for a cardiac arrest, they were all afraid it was me. One by one I was able to face my skeletons and put them aside. It took a lot of work, perseverance and prayer but I overcame it.

After the episode whenever we went away on vacation where we left the state, I could feel myself starting to breathe heavy, sigh a lot and feel my pulse speed up. Why? Because I was out of my comfort zone, I was afraid something might happen and I'd be too far away from my lifeline.

Mayo Clinic is my umbilical cord, my lifeline. They have saved my life more than one time over the years. I have a great appreciation for the skills of their doctors and nursing staff. I have discovered that we can't put ourselves in glass bubbles though, waiting for what-ifs of life to happen. I decided I was not going to live my life being afraid or with regrets.

I was getting my life back on track when the panic attacks started coming more frequently. I was walking in the mall with a friend around the early part of 1995. We would meet there every morning at around eight. Then we would do our laps and go home feeling refreshed as well as good about the fact that we had solved world problems during those early morning treks.

This one morning we were supposed to meet at our usual time. While I sat in my van waiting for my friend to arrive I started getting a feeling of claustrophobia and the walls were closing in on me. I started my usual heavy breathing and sighing routine, I was restless and getting very anxious. I had to get out of the van and walk around it to get myself calmed down. Once I felt like I was somewhat under control I got into my vehicle and headed for home.

I called my friend on my way home and told her what was happening and that I couldn't make it that day. I was so rattled by the ordeal that I called Jeff at work crying about the incident. I got his usual, "Don't be ridiculous" speech. He always tells me it is in my head, I shouldn't be nervous about this, but I just couldn't help myself.

I was finding out more and more that other than going to work I didn't want to leave the sanctuary I had built for myself, my home. I felt more comfortable there than anywhere. This is called agoraphobia, a fear of leaving the home or sanctuary that you have made for yourself. There have been documented cases where people have not left their homes for years. I didn't seem to want to go anywhere or do anything outside of my domain.

My next outing was to the dentist and while the hygienist was cleaning my teeth I evidently started bleeding from my gums. She kept rinsing my mouth again and again but it wouldn't stop. Her next comment was, "Boy this just doesn't want to quit bleeding." That threw me into a tailspin; I did everything I could to stay seated and not run out of the building screaming. I thought for sure that the devil had returned. I was able to maintain my composure until I left, then I came unglued. I cried and cried. Oh, the things that went racing through my mind were: another

207

relapse, death, perhaps a different type of cancer, you name it. I ran the gambit on myself in the two miles home from the dentist's office.

I ran in the house called Jeff and told him that I thought I was losing my mind. I told him what had happened and then told him I needed some kind of counseling. He agreed, so I went surfing through the yellow pages for therapists. I was able to locate one that could see me the next morning. I'm not quite sure how I made it through that evening at work. I arrived the next morning for my appointment early. I didn't want to be late and I truly wanted to find the source of the panic attacks and get rid of them.

I ended up doing a lot of crying in that first session. I guess I learned how to be stoic in my early years all too well. After my brother died when I was young I rode on that damn float in the Fourth of July parade in our hometown. I was supposed to smile and wave at the people. So at the age of nine I learned how to disallow my feelings and shelf them so to speak in. Being human and adult, we are all taught that we are to hold everything in which could send you to the nuthouse. Well you can apply this to about any of the emotions we as humans feel. I must agree, when my brother died I held all my emotions at bay.

My therapist told me I was suffering from post-traumatic stress disorder, "an anxiety disorder characterized by an acute emotional response to a traumatic event or situation involving severe environmental stress, as a natural disaster, airplane crash, serious automobile accident, military combat, and physical torture. Symptoms of the condition include recurrent, intrusive recollections or nightmares, diminished responsiveness to the external world, hyper alertness or an exaggerated startle response, sleep disturbances, irritability, memory impairment, difficulty in concentrating, depression, anxiety, headaches and vertigo," according to the definition from *Mosby's Medical Dictionary*. I was and still am experiencing some of these symptoms. I still watched my back for those men with the little white coats.

I was able to go through the cancer problems fairly well, but

I was affected by the cardiac arrest, it was evidently the straw that broke the camel's back. I was supposed to start allowing my feelings to come out, not to shut them off like a switch. But I should limit the time of wallowing in pity, or some other emotion I was feeling. If I felt like crying then cry, but tell myself I will only cry for ten minutes. Then I should move on, I needed to learn how to feel the emotions I had.

We started working through some things and wound up digging into my past. There are many things from my childhood that I have repressed in my memory for so long that it was uncomfortable trying to uncover them. Some psychologists say, "we should not carry our past around like monkeys on our backs, that we should let it go! We need to learn from it and let it go." Some of the cobwebs up in my attic I felt needed to stay there. So after three months of therapy I decided to let it go. Besides, I felt we were accomplishing nothing, I was learning nothing, so it was time to move on.

If I could say anything about that time I think it would be that I started to get more depressed digging into my past. I had no desire to become a blithering idiot. Digging in the past was not only painful, but I didn't find much use in forcing memories that I have forgotten for so long to be brought out. I had enough on my plate in the present, I felt that I didn't need to go excavating, I would let it go, the past was going to stay in the past.

I went for a different approach; I visited with our family doctor who explained that it was the chemistry of my brain that was lacking an ingredient, serotonin that acts as a neurotransmitter. It helps to get the messages through. He told me that I needed to start some medication to put this all back in line again, an antidepressant. I thought to myself why not, most of my relatives were on them. It couldn't hurt? I do need to give credit where credit is due though. The therapist did help me through a very painful time, so with behavior modification she taught me how to deal with my panic attacks.

I guess I was trying to win the mother of the year award. I did everything for my children and husband that I could to make their lives better. I was mistaking my guilt for being sick for love. Or perhaps it would be better to say that I was throwing myself into my family almost having a choke hold on them. I couldn't do enough; I was driving them and myself close to insanity. I once again started running in circles chasing my tail.

What do you do when you are already stressed out and on the edge of insanity? That is when I decided to go back to school and get my bachelor's degree in nursing. Not enough stress you ask?

The Vice President of Nursing that we had at our hospital at the time was truly an education buff. Most of the nurses who worked at the hospital were ADNs, the two-year registered nurse graduates. He encouraged most of us to go back and get our four-year degrees, which would give us a BSN. There weren't many BSNs at the time; the hospital was willing to grant education loans to the staff who wanted to go back to school.

The loans were to be paid off by years of service. So for every two thousand dollars you received, you were expected to work one year at the hospital. Seeing as most of us that were there were there because our husbands and families were established in the community and we wouldn't be leaving anyway. The deal sounded good…almost too good. Plus at the end you would get a one dollar an hour raise for being a four year graduate. But what I sacrificed for the almighty buck, well, was it worth it?

Each time I went to school it was because someone else was paying for my education. First I used my GI bill from my stint in the Navy. My education funds from the government were about to run out so I thought going to school was the solution to all my problems. It was funny; I took classes in the sciences and got a two-year science degree along with my two-year nursing degree.

At first I didn't know what it was that I wanted from my education. Then because I had small children at the time I needed to find a field that made sense. This was nursing. The only request I got from Jeff, who from his experiences with RNs in the Navy were not positive, was that if I went into nursing that I "better plan on being the best damn nurse I could possibly be." That put a lot on my shoulders.

I wasn't quite sure if that is what I wanted to do with the rest of my life though. I was even unsure after I graduated, got my license and was about ready to start work. It was then a nurse friend of mine reminded me, put everything into perspective, by adding those pearls of wisdom, "now you can clean up puke, poop, and pee for the rest of your life, because you have a license to do it." Boy, did that give a graduate nurse something to think about. Nonetheless I set out to be the best nurse I could be at my husband's request.

So when the window of opportunity again opened, with education being dangled in front of me like a carrot, I signed up for both the loan and classes. I truly thought that it was God talking to me and leading me in this direction.

It was during this time that I was really searching almost desperately for the answer. What was the question you ask? The question was this, God spared my life from cancer and chemotherapy related heart arrhythmias, what is it I was supposed to do with the rest of my life? That is why I thought I was supposed to get my four-year degree; the cost would be nothing out of my pocket except for books. This truly must be divine inspiration, right? It's funny how I can twist my desires into God's desires.

It is easy for all of us to start to take our lives for granted. I am no better than anyone else; this was my fault too. But our lives can become so mechanical that we miss all the little love messages that are trying to beam their way through to us. We all believe that we live in Utopia, where everything is beautiful. How does the song go, "Don't Worry be Happy"!

Chapter Thirty

ONE THING I HAVE NEGLECTED TO tell you about having Chester (my internal defibrillator), is that every year it needed to be tested. It was the battery power they needed to test, the bad news was that I had to be put under an anesthetic so they could do it. What they would do was induce the V-fib heart rhythm I originally experienced in my cardiac arrest in 1994. Chester's job was to use his power to shock me back into a normal rhythm. I had a lot of faith in him!

I did find that I would go through anxiety attacks just before I went up to the Mayo Clinic for my defibrillator testing. The checkups always went well, it was my insecurities that would send me into orbit. After the first few times it was tested, I did ease up on the anxiety a little. I could give myself cold sweats though, just going to the pacing clinic to have the nurses interrogate the device where they checked to see if Chester had been up to anything funny.

I remember in 1995 while my daughter was in high school, on the high school swim team, at a home meet she broke two school records. Chester let me know in no uncertain terms that I needed to settle down; my heart was racing so fast he zapped me. When the first zap happened I thought someone had tapped me on the shoulder so I started to turn around to see who it was and I was zapped again. The second jolt was significantly stronger than the first one and it got my attention quickly.

I was terrified, so after initially coming unglued, I went home taking to my bed. The excitement was too much for me and since Chester zapped me I was afraid of what my heart would do next. Jeff came home from the meet before Jennifer did, came into the bedroom and told me to get out of bed, "You have done enough to this family you are not going to cripple them with this." I simply complied.

Jeff is so good for me, he always keeps me grounded, even when I am to the point when I would like to do him bodily harm I still love him. I found out later that month when I went to have the device interrogated that I wasn't zapped because of an abnormal rhythm, it was because my heart rate was too fast. When I saw the doctor he decided that if I was going to attend anymore swim meets he would simply change the setting on the device, making my defibrillator to allow my heart rhythm to beat faster.

Also in 1995 as I mentioned, I went back to school which wasn't too bad, I only had four classes left to take plus the year-long required nursing courses. At first they were mostly correspondence courses, so I could work at my own pace so to speak. I found though that working on my own could be more of a hindrance than help, since procrastination is a word that is in my vocabulary. I could go to class in my "jammies" and work an hour then do some laundry, ironing or some other putsy thing I could find to do. Then I found out from my daughter that at college she would attend classes in her "jammies" in public, when she had early morning classes. This is a different generation I guess.

In 1997 was when I started my studies in an actual classroom setting. It was then I had difficulties with juggling my work, school, clinical and home. When I was in nursing school in the late eighties I only worked part-time and now in the late nineties I thought I could handle it all and worked full-time. I must have been crazy!

In order to attend some early evening classes I would work late on Tuesday and have to come back at seven in the morning on Wednesday in order to work before I went to class at five thirty. For the most part school was more manageable than I thought it would be. I was glad I was taking these classes instead of waiting much longer; it is definitely more challenging the older you are to get through all the assignments.

We had different nursing levels in our hospital. I was made a Level IV, which really didn't amount to a hill of beans. It was recognized by administration though, especially because there were very few of us. It gave me a raise, which I didn't mind, but the glitch was that I needed to finish my BSN by the year 2000. And of the Level III nurses on our unit, of which there were several, I was the closest one to that goal. So my head nurse put my name in to become a Level IV nurse, I was supposed to be looked upon as a resource person for our unit. I took part in the orientation of new nurses as they were hired, I also sat on many committees (ethics, education, quality), I also wrote, and then later revised our orientation manual. Some say I had enough on my plate with all that let alone adding more to it with school.

In 1996 Jennifer graduated from high school. She was anxious to move on to "college life"; boy do I remember being eighteen. You think that you are all grown up and can take on the world. We had an open house to celebrate her graduation. Back in the olden days, when I graduated from high school they didn't do open houses, but I didn't live in Iowa then either. Now it is very common, at least here in Mason City. It was a good celebration, and I believe Jennifer enjoyed herself as did her friends that stopped by. We displayed pictures from when she was tiny to graduation; we had examples of her artwork, essays, ribbons, trophies and her band uniform. It was fun to watch all her friends gather round and giggle when viewing her school year mementos.

At this point her goal was to become an architect at Iowa State

University. Because of her swimming abilities she was able to pick up a partial scholarship. This helped out a lot, but that meant from August until March of each year she would be at swim practice twice a day, a lot more grueling than in high school. She also had to keep up with her studies, not as easy as it seems. That summer as she prepared herself for leaving the nest, I was not looking forward to her going. We had become friends as well as mother and daughter. I was going to miss her. We enjoyed each other's company, so it was great fun to be together. But I was in school myself so I didn't have too much time for the "empty nest syndrome" to get to me. The day we dropped her off at the dorms I cried all the way home, I felt my heart was breaking.

Justin would now become the only child, Jennifer had Mom to herself when she was small and after he came along she had to share me. Well, Justin now would have the opportunity to spend his last three years in high school alone, no pesky sister around.

Things remained unchanged in our lives through the next year. The only difficulties came in the summers, when Jennifer would come home from college and think that she could continue the kind of lifestyle she had developed for herself while away. She and Justin argued more when she was back in the summers than they did when they lived under one roof as young children.

It was great to see how excited he got waiting for Jennifer to come home. His enthusiasm never lasted too long. He had gotten used to having the phone to himself (they shared a teen line). He simply got used to having her gone and for the most part he had become an only child. Spoiled is how his sister saw it, or even today still sees it. For the most part having Jennifer come home at first was hard even for Jeff and I; we all had some adjusting to do. But Jennifer who was now nineteen and a little cocky, thought that we were the ogres.

The stress was becoming overwhelming. I found myself crying a lot, I just wanted to have us be a family again, not roommates. This was difficult for me; remember I wanted to be mother of the year. As the years have past now I have finally discovered that I am no longer responsible for my children's or husband's or

215

anybody else's happiness. That revelation was so freeing. It is unfortunate that I hadn't learned this years before. I may have been able to save myself from some of the mental anguish I apparently suffered.

I admit now that we did have a tendency those first years of thinking that everything would return to "normal" whenever Jennifer came home. There's that word again. That we would just go back to being the same family we had always been. I am sure it was stifling; we weren't ready to let her grow up. She was of course still Daddy's little girl and that is how we treated her. Jennifer being Jennifer never said anything, she just moped around and let us rule over her for three months of each year. Something we would eventually pay for.

At the end of the first summer, when Jennifer headed back to school, I actually was just as happy to see her go, as she was to leave. The tension in the house had been awful, I had spoken to other mothers who said they went through the same thing, and in fact this was mild in some cases. Thinking back when Jeff and I were both nineteen we were in the United States Navy and our own. We thought we had the world by the tail too. It is part of the growing process; painful as it is they must go through it. I did tell Jeff when Jennifer was tucked away safe at school and Justin had returned to his life at the high school that I didn't want to go through another summer like that one. By Thanksgiving Justin went from hating his sister to missing her, it wouldn't last once she came home.

During her sophomore year she found a boyfriend. She was afraid to tell her father and I for fear we would go ballistic on her. We never said too much until two things occurred. One was that she decided that college was more for partying than attending classes. She thought like all underclassmen think that the professors don't take attendance anyway so they wouldn't know if she was there or not. They call this being a "freshman," that they all go through it in some respect.

The next was that she didn't actually fail classes but she had to repeat some, having to take one of them as a summer class at the local community college here at home in order to maintain her eligibility for swimming. According to NCAA rules to be able to swim and maintain her scholarship, she had to meet certain standards and she was falling short of the mark. He father made her pay for the class and books too; he said that any class she had to repeat was her financial responsibility.

The next summer was still a little tense, but nothing like the summer we had the year before. Now that she had a boyfriend she spent her time pining away for him rather than fighting with her brother. Jeff and I were not sure how we felt about the boyfriend because he was older than she was and she was sneaky now. That wasn't our child! Her father blamed this all on the boyfriend. It was hard to keep our mouths shut and at times we didn't, which only served to deepen the distance we had already made between us all.

At the end of the summer Jennifer said she didn't think she would come home in the summers anymore. She thought she would get a job and an apartment in Ames and be a grown-up. We didn't say much, which was rare, but figured a lot could happen over the next nine months.

The following spring was when I started to lose control. Jeff and Justin had been having more arguments in the evenings while I was at work, to the point that Jeff would often call me at work. Justin seemed to be out of control, he was lacking his zest for life he always had.

This was concerning, but we still hadn't seen it as too much of a problem. He was also having girl problems and that was the straw that broke the camel's back. I came home from work one night and found he and Jeff sitting in the family room with Justin sobbing into a pillow and saying, "It's no use anymore." That was my wake-up call; I noticed him and the fact that he was having problems.

Everyone was on eggshells so as to not set him off. Until one day I got a phone call from some of his friends asking if he was home yet. I asked them what they meant by that, they said he just took off in his car after the first period class; they wanted to know if he had come home. I said no, trying not to panic. The news sent Jennifer into a tailspin; she was almost hysterical. I called Jeff and the police. Just as we were giving the police his picture and description he drove up in front of the house. He had driven to Des Moines, which is approximately one hundred and twenty miles south of our home. He told us he needed to think things over. He came through the door collapsing in our arms, we told him he needed to go to the hospital, he agreed and was admitted for four days of evaluation.

We learned a lot from the experience, about our son, daughter and ourselves. Justin was diagnosed with depression, no real surprise. He needed to see a therapist, in fact we all were supposed to meet with her as a family. Justin would see her individually and then we would come in and join him. The first session we found out from Jennifer we were treating her too much like a child or young teenager and as the therapist put it "she is twenty, let her go."

Justin then piped up; he was pushing for the same privileges. The therapist quickly shut him down. We were too smothering, controlling, strict, too many rules, etc. They went on and on, the end result was that Jennifer should be able to come and go as she pleases. Out of courtesy she should tell us where she was going; but if she chose to not tell us we needed to let her alone. We needed to remember she was no longer thirteen. We hadn't realized what we had been doing.

Another little revelation was that Justin was always afraid I was going to die. He never talked about it when he was younger; he was eight when I was diagnosed with leukemia in 1989. We thought he didn't understand, so no one talked with him about his feelings. He told us that he talked to his stuffed animals in his room. He told them his fears and desires late at night. He held it all in and together for the rest of us, so we thought he was fine.

Why is it that hindsight is always 20/20? If we had known at the time he was suffering as much as he was we would've gotten him help then. Thinking back now I believe we should've all gone to therapy after my illness and subsequent cardiac arrest. We needed to release the emotions we were all feeling, including myself. Just as what happened to me when my brother was killed I was doing to my own family.

If we don't talk about it then it never happened, right? Repression was a lesson I taught both of my children all too well. We talk about it more now than we ever did, because the last two years I have been very ill and our focus was on this. There was no more *"out of sight out of mind"* sort of thing; we were living it every day.

I believe we are getting better about discussing our feelings; we still have a long way to go though. I have never quite figured out when is a good time to discuss life-threatening experiences with your family. Is this a topic of conversation at the dinner table? Could be! The children have listened to stranger things than that at an evening meal. Their mother is a nurse and their father was an EMT in his youth, and a corpsman in the United States Navy.

We all survived and have made it through the whole ordeal fairly intact. Right after Justin's episode we went to Iowa City so I could graduate from the University of Iowa. I achieved my goal! I received my bachelor's degree in nursing. It was over, all the stress of school, juggling work, clinical and home was finished. I thought that it meant that we were okay. Or were we?

Could it be possible that we were all on the edge or should we be thinking that everything could bust out all over again? For the moment we decided to take one day at a time and our motto became, just *Make Me Laugh...*

Bibliography

Funk & Wagnalls Dictionary. Grolier Limited, Canada, 1981

Mosby's Medical & Nursing Dictionary. The C.V. Mosby Company, St. Louis, Missouri, 1986

Webster's New World Dictionary. Popular Library, New York, 1974

Printed in the United States
49929LVS00003B/190-492